Studies of Brain Function, Vol. 6

Moshe Abeles

Local Cortical Circuits

An Electrophysiological Study

With 31 Figures

Springer-Verlag
Berlin Heidelberg New York 1982

Professor MOSHE ABELES
Department of Physiology
The Hebrew University-Hadassah Medical School
P.O. Box 1172
Jerusalem/Israel

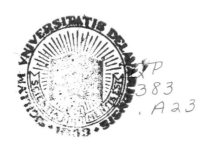

ISBN 3-540-11034-8 Springer-Verlag Berlin Heidelberg New York
ISBN 0-387-11034-8 Springer-Verlag New York Heidelberg Berlin

Library of Congress Cataloging in Publication Data
Abeles, Moshe, 1936-Local cortical circuits. (Studies of brain function ; v. 6)
Bibliography: p. Includes index.
1. Neural circuitry. 2. Cerebral cortex. 3. Action potentials
(Electrophysiology) I. Title. II. Series. [DNLM: 1. Cerebral cortex-- Analysis.
2. Cerebral cortex--Physiology. 3. Electrophysiology. W1 ST937KF v. 6 /
WL 307 A141L5]   QP383.A23   599.01'88   81-18489   AACR2

Offsetprinting: Julius Beltz, Hemsbach/Bergstr.
Binding: Konrad Triltsch, Graphischer Betrieb, Würzburg
2131/3130-543210

This work is dedicated to the memory of
J. MAGNES *my teacher, colleague and friend.*

Contents

1 Introduction

Neurophysiologists are often accused by colleagues in the physical sciences of designing experiments without any underlying hypothesis. This impression is attributable to the ease of getting lost in the ever-increasing sea of professional publications which do not state explicitly the ultimate goal of the research. On the other hand, many of the explicit models for brain function in the past were so far removed from experimental reality that they had very little impact on further research.

It seems that one needs much intimate experience with the real nervous system before a reasonable model can be suggested. It would have been impossible for Copernicus to suggest his model of the solar system without the detailed observations and tabulations of star and planet motion accumulated by the preceeding generations. This need for intimate experience with the nervous system before daring to put forward some hypothesis about its mechanism of action is especially apparent when theorizing about cerebral cortex function.

There is widespread agreement that processing of information in the cortex is associated with complex spatio-temporal patterns of activity. Yet the vast majority of experimental work is based on single neuron recordings or on recordings made with gross electrodes to which tens of thousands of neurons contribute in an unknown fashion. Although these experiments have taught us a great deal about the organization and function of the cortex, they have not enabled us to examine the spatio-temporal organization of neuronal activity in any detail.

During the last 8 years I have carried out, together with a group of gifted students (A. Ariely, Y. Assaff, R. Frostig, Y. Gottlied, Y. Hodis and E. Vaadia), a number of research projects, in which we concentrated on obtaining records from groups of neurons in the cortex.

This monograph attempts to share with the reader the insights we have gained about the interactions within small groups of neurons. Although the experimental evidence that led to these insights will be discussed in enough detail to support our conclusions, this book is not written as a technical report.

Three lines of thought are woven throughout the monograph. In the first place I have tried to describe the types of activities and interactions that are seen when several cortical neurons are studied simultaneously. It is hoped that this description will enable the reader to acquire a feeling for what goes on in a network of cortical neurons while in operation. The second theme of this work is a combination of the histology and the physiology of the cortex on a quantitative basis. Although the calculations performed are very primitive and could use refinement and extension, they do illustrate how the extensively connected network of neurons might interact to yield the observed physiological properties and they set a stage for further quantitative evaluation of the cortical network. The third idea is to state explicitly the problems and the hypotheses which are to be tested by the experiments and to discuss the expected results before the experimental results are given. The theoretical arguments are intentionally presented in black and white to make the point as explicit as possible. It is left to the reader to elaborate the intermediate cases.

This monograph was initiated in the autumn of 1978 when, following a talk at the Max Planck Institut für Biologische Kybernetik in Tübingen about interactions between neurons in the auditory cortex, Valentino Braitenberg asked me to summarize my work for *Studies of Brain Function.* I accepted this kind invitation gladly for two reasons. I thought it would be a good opportunity to review the many pieces of evidence we have collected and to try to construct a coherent picture of the functioning of the cortical network. I also thought that it would be worthwhile to write a text that would introduce the newcomer into the field of electrophysiological studies of interactions among neurons.

Meanwhile, two new ideas have reached maturity in our laboratory: The idea of organization of activity of neurons in synchronously firing groups and a statistical approach for measuring the organization of neural activity. I have exploited the opportunity given to me here to expose these ideas for the first time.

While writing the text, I had three types of readers in mind. A reader to whom cortical physiology is new, either because his main interest is in another field or because he is just starting to work on the cortex. For this type of reader I included briefly the main facts and ideas required as a baseline for understanding the text. I did assume, however, that basic properties of nerve cell morphology and physiology are known to the reader. The second type of reader I had in mind is a physiologist who is not particularly familiar with our own work but has a good knowledge of current concepts in cortical neurophysiology. This reader may wish to skip all of Chapter 2 (Techniques) and parts 1 and 2 of Chapter 3 dealing with the patterns of spontaneous activity of single neurons. The last type of reader, the proficient electrophysiologist of the cortex, may find new approaches for analysis of cortical activity in Chapter 3.3 and 3.4 and Chapter 4.5, in Chapter

7, where a new hypothesis about the coding of information in the cortex is developed and in Chapter 8, where a new technique for the analysis of organization of large populations of neurons is suggested.

This monograph does not attempt to review the vast literature covering the subjects it touches upon. It is a one-sided description of affairs, biased by my own experiments and by the prejudices and views that evolved from them. In each topic I have tried to include one or two references that would give a lead to further reading on the subject. These references are not necessarily the most significant contributions nor the most extensive reviews but are just an opening for the reader to get into the subject.

2 Techniques

This chapter summarizes in brief the extracellular recording techniques we used for recording spike activity of single nerve cells and the main methods for spike train analysis. The reader familiar with standard electrophysiological techniques may skip this chapter.

2.1 Single-Unit Recording

Whenever there is a difference in electric potential between two parts of a nerve cell there is an electric current flowing from the more positive region to the more negative region. The current flows both inside the cell and outside the cell in opposite directions. The flow of current through the outside medium is associated with a potential gradient through the medium which may be measured through a microelectrode located there.

The potential gradient in the extracellular volume conductors is proportional to the current density and to the specific resistance of the extracellular medium.

Slow changes of the membrane potential tend to spread over larger distances than spikes due to two factors:
1. The cell membrane has higher impedance for slow waves and therefore adjacent parts of a neuron cannot maintain passively a large steady difference in their transmembrane potential (the equivalent length constant for slow waves is large); by contrast, spikes contain higher frequencies which are short-circuited by the capacitive nature of the membrane (the equivalent length constant for high frequencies is small). Thus, when the soma is depolarized synaptically, the cell body, together with the large dendrites, acts as a current *sink* while the remote dendrites (several hundreds of micrometers away) may act as a current *source*. The current flowing between such a remote *source* and *sink* will spread laterally over a large distance; whereas if an action potential develops in the cell's body the large dendrites become *sources*, thereby limiting the range of current spread in the extracellular volume conductor.

2. The extracellular space of the cortex is not a homogenous volume conductor but is packed with cell processes covered by lipid membranes conducting low frequencies poorly. This factor may also cause the low frequency slow waves to spread over greater distances.

The result is that when a metal microelectrode is pushed into the cortex we see a mixture of slow waves (very similar to what one sees when recording the electrocortiogram with macroelectrodes) and spike-like events.

Figure 1A is a schematic diagram of the electric field around a neuron during an action potential. A metal microelectrode is also drawn, for comparison of size.

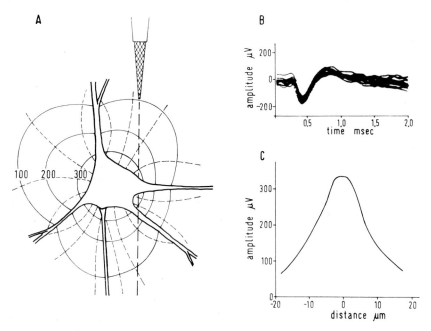

Fig. 1 A-C. Single unit recording with extracellular microelectrode.
A Imaginary view of a pyramidal neuron when an action potential is developing in its soma. Lines of current flow (*broken lines*) and equipotential lines (*full lines*). When a metal microelectrode (*top right*) insulated all the way to the tip is moved close to the cell we may see a spike-like event. **B** Superposition of many such spikes. As long as the electrode is in a fixed position they all look alike. **C** Changes in the height of the peak of the spike with changes in the electrode position

In standard experiments we filtered out most of the slow waves and were left with spike-like pulses and high frequency (100-10,000 Hz) noise. On close examination of the large spikes we usually observe the same spike shape repeatedly (Fig. 1B). Under such circumstances we say that these spikes represent the activity of a single unit — presumably a single neuron. This assumption is further strengthened by the observation that as the electrode is moved a few micrometers up or down the spike shapes may increase or decrease in amplitude but they remain similar to each other. The amplitude of a spike of given shape varies continuously with electrode position (unless we happen to injure the cell or one of its processes) and can be recorded on the average over a range of 30 μm (Fig. 1C).

We assume that all the information carried from one nerve cell to the others is coded in the times of spikes traversing along its axon. Our interest, therefore, centers on the times of occurrence of spikes rather than on the shapes of individual spikes. The detection techniques described in the next section are designed to convert the spike train recorded from a given cell into a sequence of times of occurrences.

2.2 Multi-Unit Analysis

In practice several spike shapes may be recorded from a given electrode position during any period of time. Some researchers work on that "mixed" activity as it is, stating that they are dealing with multi-unit activity. Others wishing to study a single unit may move the electrode carefully up or down until one of the spike shapes becomes considerably bigger than the others and may work on this one alone. We wish to study several single units simultaneously, in order to learn something about the interactions among units in localized cortical neural networks.

For that purpose we developed a special pattern detector (P.D.D. 256 Yissum, Jerusalem) which detects automatically each spike as it occurs, compares it with two templates, and represents it as a dot whose coordinates are a measure of the degree of match between the recorded spike and the templates[1]. This method is illustrated in Fig. 2.

The two templates with which each spike is compared are shown in Fig. 2A. At the point of optimal match a dot is plotted. When the same spike shape appears repeatedly a cluster of points is generated. By putting windows around the clusters the various shapes may be separated from each other. Four clusters are marked in Fig. 2B and the actual wave shapes in each of these clusters is shown in Fig. 2C. Cluster 1 corresponds to a mixture of small spikes and noise, while clusters 2, 3, and 4 correspond to three different single units.

---

1 The degree of match between a recorded shape R(t) and a template S(t) is given by their inner product $\int_0^2 R(t)S(t)dt$ and is equivalent to the Euclidian projection of the vector R(t) on the vector S(t).

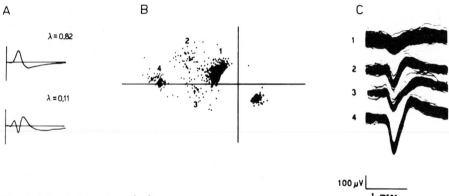

Fig. 2 A-C. Multi-unit analysis.
A Two orthonormal templates used to detect and characterize the spike. **B** Representation of 15 s of activity. Each spike is rß epresented by a *dot* whose coordinates are proportional to the degree of matching of the spike to the two templates. Windows were placed over four clusters. Each time a dot fell in one of the windows we could see also the actual spike shape that was represented by the dot. **C** The spike shapes represented by the *dots* in the four clusters. Cluster *1* contains noise and small spikes. Clusters *2, 3,* and *4* contain each single unit

   With this method it is fairly easy to obtain three or four single units from the same electrode, by searching the cortex carefully up to seven single units could be obtained from such recordings. All the units obtained with this method are close to the electrode tip; on the average we expect them to be within 30 μm from each other although occasionally they may be as far as 100 μm apart.

   (A more detailed description of this method may be found in Friedman 1968, Abeles and Goldstein 1977).

2.3 Limitations of Our Recording Technique

   The metal microelectrodes have exposed tips of 10-20 μm. Such electrodes have two important properties: their impedance is low (0.3-1 MΩ at 1000 Hz) and they average the electric fields along their exposed surface. These properties favor the recording of small potentials which extend over large distances. We can record small potentials because the electrode has low noise, but the potential must not fall off too steeply, or else it is averaged out by the length of the electrode tip. This type of electrode is selective for electric fields set up near the cell soma. Other types of electrodes in use are small tip Tungsten microelectrode and micropipettes, which have high noise and record from a point in the volume conductor. These characteristics favor picking up of potentials from axons (Kiang 1965) or perhaps from dendrites, whose high potentials extend only over short distances (see Rall 1962, for a theoretical analysis of spread of potentials around soma and dendrites).

The experimental procedures used to discover the single unit introduced additional sampling bias. In a typical experiment the electrode is pushed through the tissue until a well-defined single unit or several units are seen. The probability of tapping the activity of such single units is proportional to the cross-section area of the region in which extracellular spike may be recorded. The transmembrane action potential is almost the same in all neurons, therefore, the extent of the extracellular field will depend mainly on the size and geometry of the dendrites. Usually cells with large somata have thick dendrites extending over large distances and would therefore have large extracellular fields. The somata of small cells in the auditory cortex are about 8 μm in diameter and the biggest are around 20 μm. On a first-order approximation one would assume that the cell size is proportional to the extent of the extracellular electric field, therefore, an electrode is 6 (20/8 squared) times more likely to encounter the largest cells. However, the small cortical cells are numerous while the largest ones are scarce and concentrated in the deep layers. Hence, our sample is biased in favor of the big cells, but contains both small and large cells, as may be seen from comparing Fig. 3A to Fig. 3B.

The last factor affecting our sampling is the firing rate of the cortical cells. Cells with high firing rates are more likely to be noticed as the electrode is advanced through the brain. Cells with low firing rates are easily noticed when the recorded spike is very large but will generally pass unnoticed when it is small and mixed with several other spikes firing at higher rates. Some cortical cells may not fire at all and those are not detected by the single-unit technique.

In our experiments no special stimulus is given when we search for units. The probability of our detecting units depends, therefore, on their spontaneous rate of firing (Fig. 3C). In cases where the researcher applies stimuli while searching for units, the unit sample is biased in favor of the responding units. This type of bias is probably stronger when the experimental animal is anesthetized, even if lightly. Under anesthesia most cells have reduced firing rates and many cells cease to respond (Goldstein 1968, Chap. 2).

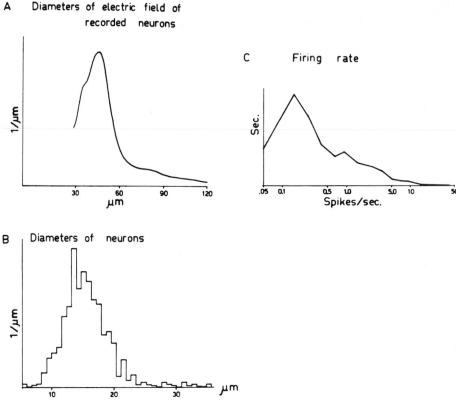

Fig. 3 A-C. Properties of neurons in the auditory cortex of cat
A Probability-density function of diameters of recordable electric fields of neurons.
B Probability-density function of neuron diameter. The abscissa of **A** is scaled so that
the recordable field of each cell is plotted just above the corresponding cell size in **B**.
C Probability-density function of the rate of firing of recorded units in the nonanesthe-
tized nonstimulated cat.

2.4 Analysis of Spike Trains by Renewal Density

When a single unit activity is detected, we represent it by the time of
occurrences of the spikes. Such an abstraction, dealing only with the epochs
of neural discharge, is justified by the assumption that all the information
which traverses the axon is contained in the time series of epochs. We also
assume that spikes in the cortical neuron are generated by a process similar
to that worked out by Eccles for the motoneuron in the spinal cord (Eccles
1957), namely that incoming impulses at the dendritic tree and the soma
induce conductivity changes setting up currents which add up more or less
passively. These currents change the transmembrane potential of the cell

body. One or more points of the neuron have a low threshold for spike generation. When the threshold at such a trigger zone is reached a spike is generated, it invades the whole of the cell body and propagates along the axon to affect other neurons.

Although the functional role of the spike train is to transmit information through the neural network, we may use it as a tool for studying the internal neural mechanisms governing spike generation. For instance, if one neuron excites a second neuron synaptically, the probability of firing of the other, post-synaptic, neuron will increase. The time course of this increase in probability depends in some way on the shape of the post-synaptic potential generated by the exciting cell. Hence by studying the firing patterns of a cell we can learn about the neurophysiological mechanisms of the spike generation.

These arguments may be summarized by stating that studies of spike trains can be conducted from two points of view: (1) What is the code of information carried by the spike train? (2) What are the neurophysiological mechanisms underlining the recorded spike train?

Most of the following discussion is related to the second question. Only in later chapters as we encounter phenomena that cannot be explained in a simple way by the known anatomy and physiology of the cortex shall we turn our attention back to the question of information coding.

While studying neurophysiological mechanisms we shall assume that the spike train represents a realization of a *renewal process* (Cox 1970). In such a process the probability of an event (spike in our case) depends only on the time elapsed since the last event (and not on the events prior to it). The assumption that a spike train can be treated statistically as a renewal process is justified by the observation that each spike resets the transmembrane potential of the neuron's body. In this way all the synaptic processes that preceded the spike are "forgotten" and the depolarization has to be rebuilt in order to reach threshold. However, one has to bear in mind that transmembrane potential resetting occurs only in the soma and large dendrites, and does not affect considerably the remote dendrites. Therefore, the renewal process is just a first-order statistical approximation to the spike train. In this monograph I shall concentrate on one mode of representing the data, the representation by renewal density. This type of representation plots the firing rate of a nerve cell as a function of time elapsed from a specific, well-defined event. The idea behind this approach is that the firing rate of the cell represents the excitability of the cell. The higher the excitability, the higher the firing rate. Although the relation is not linear it is a monotonous function and the exact relation may be worked out (see Sampath and Srinivasan 1977, Holden 1976 for extensive reviews of such relations).

The event from which we start to measure time may be quite different in various experiments. It may be the time at which an external stimulus was given. In this case the renewal density plots the variations of firing rate triggered by the stimulus. This is the most popular way of studying single units and is best known to physiologists by the name of Peri Stimulus Time Histogram (PSTH); Fig. 13 illustrates such graphs.

The event used to reset the starting point may be the neuron's own firing. In this case the graph shows the rate of firing of a neuron as a function of time elapsed from the firing of that neuron (e.g., Fig. 4). This type of curve is commonly called the autocorrelation or autocovariance curve (Perkel et al. 1967a), but the proper statistical name is renewal density (Cox 1970). I shall use here the term *auto-renewal density* to be differentiated from the *cross-renewal-density* which depicts the firing rate of one cell as a function of time elapsed from the firing of another cell (e.g., Fig. 7). The cross-renewal density curve is most familiar to physiologists under the name of cross-correlation (or cross-covariance) curve (Perkel et al. 1967b). The most complex renewal density with which we shall deal here is the *triple-renewal density* in which the firing rate of one cell is plotted as a function of time elapsed from the times of firing of two other cells[2].

All these types of renewal density curves will be discussed briefly at the appropriate point in the text. A detailed description of the statistical techniques used for estimating these curves may be found in Perkel et al. 1967 a, b, Perkel et al. 1975, Abeles 1982.

---

2 The term renewal density should be properly used only when the event used to reset time resets also all processes that control the firing times of the neuron to some initial conditions. For recorded neural activity we do not know whether this is the case. Nevertheless we preserve here the term *renewal density* (rather than *correlation*) to indicate that our graphs estimate the instantaneous firing rate of the neurons as a function of time elapsed from the retriggering event

3 The Spontaneous Firing of Cortical Neurons

3.1 Patterns of Firing

As one looks at the spike train of a cortical neuron no obvious order can be seen. The apparently random spike train may, however, contain some hidden patterns. Searching for such patterns is quite difficult. The patterns of firing that one looks for depend largely on the type of model that one has in mind. On the one hand, one may assume that the spike train is like a Morse code in which each sequence of intervals has a specific meaning. On the other hand, the average rate of firing over some time interval may be the only significant feature of the spike train.

The Morse code type is attractive in its ability to assign to each axon a high capacity for transmitting information (Abeles and Lass 1975). However, it would usually take very complex neuronal machinery to generate and decipher a precise Morse code of that sort. So far there has been no experimental support for the existence of such Morse-type code in the spike trains of cortical cells.

The spike rate code is attractive in that temporal summation of post-synaptic potentials will serve to translate the rate of firing of the presynaptic cell into a graded excitatory or inhibitory influence on the post-synaptic cell. In the periphery it is often observed that intensity of a given stimulus is coded in the rate of firing of nerve cells. In the somato-sensory system there is a good match between the psychophasical discriminability of stimulus intensities and the information content of the firing rate of primary sensory afferents. In both psychophysical experiments and electrophysiological recording the amount of information transmitted is a little less than three bits per stimulus (e.g., Werner and Mountcastle 1965, Miller 1963). This does not mean that the temporal structure of the spike train has no relevance. In the auditory system, for example, the timing of spikes coming from both ears is essential for localizing a sound source in space. Moreover, there is accumulating evidence that at moderate and high intensities of sound the temporal code in the auditory nerve fibers becomes the cue for analysis of complex sound (e.g., Evans 1978, Young and Sachs 1979).

A convenient way for revealing internal structure in the spike train is by computing the auto-renewal density. This graph is obtained by the following procedure: After each spike time is divided into contiguous bins; each succeeding spike adds one to the bin corresponding to its time of occurrence. The procedure is repeated again and again until all the spikes are exhausted (Perkel et al. 1967a). This process is similar to the way of constructing a Peri Stimulus Time Histogram except that in the case of auto-renewal density the spikes themselves are treated as the stimulus. When the procedure is completed the counts are converted to rate by dividing the number of spikes by the duration of measurement within each bin — $N\Delta t$; where N is the number of spikes that triggered the counting process and Δt is the bin size (Abeles 1982). As a result we obtain graphs as in Fig. 4. The abscissa represents the time elapsed from the firing of a spike by that neuron; the ordinate represents the rate of firing. Thus, the renewal density curve shows the fluctuations of the firing rate of a cell as a function of time which elapsed since previous firing.

A renewal density curve derived from a completely random point process such as the disintegration of radioactive isotope (Poisson process) would in theory be flat at a level corresponding to the average discharge rate. However, due to the limited time of measurement the measured renewal density is bound, in practice, to fluctuate around this average rate. The limits within which 99% of the curve derived from an equivalent Poisson process would fall are indicated together with each curve.

The auto-renewal density of all cortical neurons deviates from the random Poisson process in the first few milliseconds (Fig. 4A). The initial low rate of firing is attributed to the refractory periods (absolute and relative); each spike is followed by a period of low excitability, therefore the firing rate immediately after a spike is lower. This refractoriness lasts a few milliseconds, although occasionally it may last as long as 100 ms. Very few cortical neurons show oscillatory activity in the nonanesthetized state. Figure 4C illustrates a rare case in which a unit in the auditory cortex of a paralyzed cat showed some rhythmicity at a frequency of 20 per minute. This period coincides with that of the respiration pump which maintained the cat. It is quite likely that the slight noise made by the flow of air through the tracheal cannula led to the periodic stimulation of that auditory neuron. In most of 400 cortical units studied we did not find any conspicuous fluctuations of the auto-renewal density beyond the initial 100 ms and therefore we decided to measure the renewal density up to a maximal delay of 500 ms (Fig. 4B).

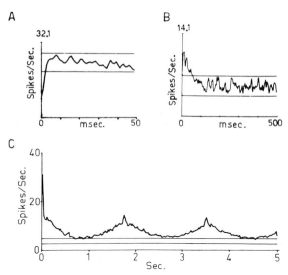

Fig. 4 A-C. Auto-renewal densities for cortical neurons.
A On expanded scale very fast processes may be seen. In this case the refractoriness of
the cell is evident. **B** A typical renewal density for a cortical neuron in an unanesthetized
animal. **C** On compressed time scale slow-processes may be seen. Here the unit fired
rhythmically at the rate of the respiration pump

3.2 Neural Mechanisms

The shape of the autorenewal density function of a cell reflects two
factors — internal excitability changes after each spike generated by the
cell and the pattern of activity of those neurons which excite or inhibit
that cell.

The most common internal excitability changes are the absolute and relative refractory periods; the excitability changes generated by *after-potentials*
following each spike will also affect the shape of the auto-renewal density
curve. Cells having pacemaker potentials have periodic auto-renewal density
functions.

The effect of the refractory periods was seen in every auto-renewal density function examined by us as a depression of firing rate during the first
few milliseconds. A prolonged depression such as should be generated by
an after-hyperpolarization was seen only in 7% of the units studied. In
most neurons each spike is followed by a phase of increased potassium permeability accompanied by after-hyperpolarization. It is unlikely that 93%
of the cortical neurons do not show this process. We must assume then that
the effects of the after-hyperpolarization are masked by some other factors.
These factors will be discussed later.

The auto-renewal density function is very sensitive to periodic changes in the firing rate, so that even small periodic changes embedded in high random noise would be expected to show up. Our inability to find such periodic changes (except for the few cases entrained by the respiration pump) indicates that cortical neurons do not contain internal pacemaker mechanisms.

The spontaneous ongoing activity of cortical neurons depends on inputs arriving to the region through the underlying white matter. On the average, over 99% of the input to the cortex comes from the cortex (locally or from other cortical areas, Braitenberg 1978a). We must, therefore, conclude that the activity we record when no specific stimulus is given to the animal is due to internal cortical mechanisms in which neurons are being excited by other neurons, then in turn excite other neurons, and so on.

What are the modes of activity that can be expected to occur in such self-exciting networks? Three distinct modes come to mind: random, periodic, and bursting.

Random Poisson-like firing is expected when the firing times of different cells are uncorrelated. Under these conditions the multitude of EPSP's and IPSP's evoked in any given neuron summate to a fluctuating transmembrane potential looking like white noise but filtered through the cell membrane time constants. This fluctuating wave would exceed the threshold level at random times and therefore give rise to a random spike train. Such a model is consistent with the notion that the superposition of many independent point processes adds up to a random Poisson process (Cox 1970). Models of this type have been discussed extensively by Sampath and Srinivasan (1977). However, when different cells have correlated firing, superposition of their spike trains may add up to some nonrandom patterns.

Periodic firing could be generated by a single cell, as discussed earlier, but could also be due to reverbrations in neural circuits. Such reverberations may traverse well-defined anatomical circuits carrying excitation in closed loops, or may also travel in dynamically changing pathways in which excitation may follow complex multisynaptic routs changing from time to time. In such cases each cycle of the reverberation may traverse a different chain of neurons. Both types of circuits were postulated in the cortex (Lorente de No 1949, Hebb 1949), and were assumed to be responsible for carrying memory and for information processing. We were, therefore, puzzled by our inability to find periodicities in the firing of cortical units.

We looked for periodicities in two types of preparations: the nonanesthetized, muscle-relaxed cat and the behaving monkey. Before proceeding to describe these experiments a word of explanation about the experimental animals is required.

As will become evident in the following sections, it was essential to work with unanesthetized animals. However, at the early stages of our work we could not record from behaving animals. Therefore, most of the experiments were carried out on muscle-relaxed cats. In this type of preparation it is very important to take care that the animal does not feel any pain. For that purpose, the animal was operated on under deep surgical anesthesia and all wounds were treated by local anesthetics. The recordings started only after the anesthesia faded out (24-36 h after it was induced). By examination of the EEG, the blood pressure, and the size of pupils, it seemed that the animal was sleeping lightly. Any unusual sound produced transient arousal from which the animal went back to its "sleeping" state within few seconds. Presumably, the animal did not feel pain or else it would have stayed aroused (see Goldstein et al. 1968, for more details on this type of preparation).

In the behaving monkeys too, all surgical procedures were carried out under deep anesthesia. However, the microelectrodes were introduced into the cortex only few days later. From the monkey's behavior it was apparent that the electrode penetration and the recording were not aversive, as it continued to come willingly and sit in the restraining chair in which the experiment was carried out almost daily for several weeks.

In an early set of experiments Dr. Y. Gottlieb examined the effect of barbiturates on the firing patterns of cortical neurons. In the nonanesthetized, muscle-relaxed cat he recorded the spontaneous activity of neurons and then injected low (subanesthetic) doses of barbiturate. With the appearance of barbiturate spindles in the EEG, the units started to fire periodically at the same frequency as the EEG spindles and in a time-locked fashion to the EEG waves. This type of periodicity seems to be specifically brought about by the drug, and was not seen during spontaneous EEG spindling in the nonanesthetized state.

In a different series of experiments Y. Gottlieb trained a Baboon to perform the following short-term memory task. The monkey heard two tone peeps separated by 1 s of silence. It was trained to press one button if the two tones had the same pitch and another button if they were different. Within each session 16 tone combinations were used, the frequencies were changed from day to day, forcing the monkey to use short-term memory in order to perform the task correctly. Correct responses were reinforced by delivering 0.1 cc of sweetened water. With adequate training the monkey could perform this task with a 95% success rate over several hundreds of trials per session. If the water spout (through which the reward for correct performance was delivered) was taken away, the monkey immediately stopped responding and the stimuli; that period served as control. When the water spout was reinstalled the monkey immediately began to respond again.

After training, the monkey was anesthetized, the skull was opened and a recording chamber was mounted over the hole. After recovery a microelectrode could be inserted into the auditory cortex through the chamber and into the brain so that single-unit recordings could be made while the monkey performed the task.

About 30% of the units picked up in the auditory cortex showed different patterns of firing during the interval between the first and second tones when the responding and control periods were compared. Figure 5A and B shows the firing rate of such a unit during the performance of the task (full line) and during the control period (dotted line). In the performing state the unit maintained a high firing rate throughout the interval between the two tone pips, despite the abscene of any external stimulus at that time. This maintained high rate of firing is not due to reverberation in loops of fixed length, since the auto-renewal density of the cell does not show any sign of rhythmic activity (Fig. 5C and D). Indeed none of the 40 units showing sustained changes of firing rates between the two stimuli showed any sign of reverberation.

We conclude that periodic reverberation is not a mode of activity in the awake and functioning cortex.

The last form of organization of activity that will be considered here is bursting. When a nerve cell is depolarized above the threshold level for an extended period it is likely to fire with a burst of spikes; when these spikes arrive at the next, post-synaptic, neuron they are likely to elicit there a prolonged depolarization which may in turn produce a burst of spikes, and so on. Thus, if most of the neurons in a network are exciting each other by bursts of activity, it is likely that the bursting pattern will maintain itself throughout the network.

Neurons whose activity is organized in bursts are occasionally found in the cortex. Many physiologists think that such bursts of activity are produced by injury of the cell. While most injured cells do fire in bursts it is not known whether the converse is also true. At any rate, most cells do not fire in well-defined bursts, but fire single spikes with a slight tendency to bursting. The initial hump of the renewal density as shown in Fig. 4B is present in most (70%) of the renewal densities studied. The hump indicates that a cell shortly after firing a spike is more likely to fire again. However, the area under the hump is usually small, and amounts to about 0.3 spikes. This means that on the average each spike is followed by 0.3 spikes more than would be expected for a random Poisson process. Is this slight tendency toward bursting enough to support itself as a mode of activity or is there also some internal neuronal mechanism to generate this pattern of firing?

There is a need for a quantitative analysis to investigate the possibility that a slight tendency for neuron activity to occur in bursts would be per-

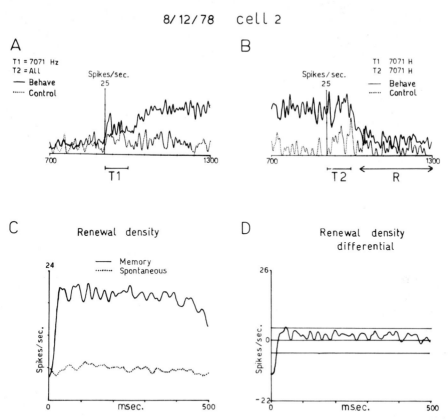

8/12/78   cell 2

Fig. 5 A-D. Activity of a single unit in auditory cortex during a short-term memory task
A, B Rate of firing during the task. Tone 1 was one of four frequencies, it was followed
by 1 s of silence and then by Tone 2 which was composed of one of four frequencies.
A The effect of the first tone *(T1)* on the firing rate of the unit. This graph is constructed from all the cases in which T1 was 7071 Hz. **B** The effect of the second tone *(T2)*
on the firing rate of the unit. This graph is constructed from all the cases in which both
T2 and T1 were 7071 Hz. In the control period *(dotted line)* the monkey did not respond.
During the behavior period *(solid line)* the monkey pressed the left botton if tone 1 was
equal to tone 2 and the right button if they were different. The range of response latency is marked as *R*. **C** Auto-renewal density derived from firing during behavior. The
solid line is the renewal density during the 1 s of silence which followed the presentation
of T1 (7071 Hz); it represents the pattern of firing when the unit "remembers" the
7071 Hz. The *dotted line* is the renewal density during the pauses between trials; it represents the pattern of "spontaneous" activity. **D** A differential auto-renewal density
in which the possible direct effects of the stimulus were eliminated. None of the auto
renewals showed any sign of reverberation. (Figure provided by courtesy of Dr. Y. Gottlieb)

petuated within the cortical network. But even if such a mode of activity
cannot maintain itself, there exists an alternative neuronal mechanism that
could account for the initial hump in the autorenewal density functions.

As mentioned earlier, the auto-renewal density function is expected to show a prolonged depression during the first 10 to 100 ms, owing to the increased potassium permeability that follows each spike. In addition, the spike sets up large currents obliterating any passive depolarization that preceded it. Thus the EPSP's must build up depolarization until a threshold is reached — the spike will then reset all the remaining effects of the previous EPSP's, it will be followed by increasing potassium permeability that hyperpolarize the soma and a new buildup of depolarization from its current value toward the threshold takes place. Although this description of events is accurate for the soma and large dendrites, where the currents set up by the spike erase all the passive remainders of the preceding synaptic currents, the duration of the spike is too short to invade the remote dendrites passively, so that in these regions the slow synaptic potentials continue past the time of firing at the soma. In this process excitation derived from the soma and large dendrites is reset by every action potential, while excitation derived from remote dendrites follows very much the time course of the depolarization at these dendrites and is affected only slightly by an action potential at the soma.

When these processes are considered, it seems likely that the initial hump in the auto-renewal density curve may reflect excitatory processes at remote dendritic sites, indicating that these processes control the timing of many of the spikes generated by the neuron. The shape of the hump will correspond to the shape of the EPSP at the remote dendrites as seen in the soma. Indeed it has recently been argued that due to the large input impedance of small dendrites synaptic currents generate there very large voltage changes which are quite effective at the soma.

In summary, then, the firing pattern of neurons is fairly random except for the effect of the refractory periods and a slight tendency to bursting which may be accounted for by assuming that excitation from remote dendrites plays a sizeable role in eliciting spikes.

3.3 Membrane Potential, Threshold, and Excitability

In this section we will attempt to gain a better insight as to how the transmembrane potential is related to the excitability of the cell. One's intuitive feeling is that the difference between the transmembrane potential and the threshold potential is the dominating factor for relating these two variables, but one has to consider also how hard it is to shift the membrane potential from its current value toward the threshold. This latter factor is related to the conductivity of the membrane which may change considerably without much change in the membrane potential itself.

If we wish to combine these factors, distance from membrane potential to threshold and the effect of synaptic currents on the membrane potential, and to relate them to the spontaneous rate of firing of the nerve cell we may view the membrane potential fluctuations as in Fig. 6A.

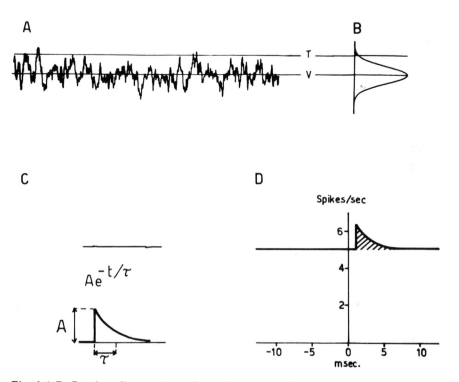

Fig. 6 A-D. Random fluctuations of membrane potential
A Hypothetical transmembrane fluctuations of a cortical neuron around some mean value V Once in a while the potential is carried to the threshold level T and then a spike is generated. 0.25 s of activity are displayed. **B** A Gaussian bell turned on its side represents the probability density of the membrane potential. The rate of firing of the neuron is proportional to the probability of the membrane potential to be above the threshold T. **C** We assume that all the postsynaptic potentials have these shapes. On the top trace one EPSP and one IPSP are drawn to scale with the transmembrane fluctuations in **A.** Below is a blown-up shape of the EPSP. Summation of many thousands of these at random time generate the wave form in **A. D** The expected effect of a single standard EPSP on the firing rate of the cell

The spontaneously fluctuating membrane potential looks very much like an electrocorticogram (ECoG), containing mostly low frequencies and having roughly a Gaussian distribution of amplitudes. Occasionally, when the potential exceeds the threshold level a spike is generated. The firing rate represents the frequency of that event. We assume that each spike corresponds to 1 ms during which the membrane potential is above threshold. Hence, the membrane potential of a nerve cell firing at 5 per second (the average spontaneous rate in our studies) has a probability of $5/1000 = 0.005$ of being above threshold. In this way we can compute the probability of the cell's transmembrane potential to be above the threshold from the firing rate of the cell. Conversely, if we know the probability of the transmembrane potential to be above threshold we can compute the firing rate of the cell. This probability is represented in Fig. 6B by the area of the probability density curve above the threshold value and it is determined by the vertical distance T between the threshold and the mean.

The area of the tail in the standard Gaussian bell is 0.005 when T is removed 2.58 standard deviations from the mean. This distance of threshold from the mean (expressed in standard deviations) is the controlling variable for the rate of firing. We shall refer to this distance as T/σ (T for threshold, σ for standard deviation). In Fig. 6B the distance T/σ is 2.3, meaning that the probability of the transmembrane potential being above threshold at any point in time is 0.011. The firing rate of this cell is expected to be $1000 \times 0.011 = 11$ per second.

To illustrate this point let us now see how various influences on the cell would affect the T/σ distance and thereby change its firing rate.

a) Synaptic depolarization brings the average membrane potential closer to threshold, thereby decreasing T and hence T/σ decreases too. The depolarization will increase the firing rate of the cell (as long as it is not too big to produce a change in threshold too).

b) Synaptic hyperpolarization moves the membrane potential away from the threshold, thereby increasing T/σ. This process of course reduces the firing rate of the cell.

c) Similar changes can be produced by neural modulators which might alter the threshold voltage rather than the average membrane potential.

d) An increase in the conductivity of the membrane to chloride ions will reduce the firing rate of the nerve cell without affecting the threshold or the average membrane potential. It does this by decreasing the range of fluctuations of the transmembrane potential, that is it decreases the standard deviation σ of the fluctuations, thereby increasing T/σ.

To summarize, all of the factors which are known to affect excitability and firing rate will affect the T/σ ratio in a consistent manner. Increased T/σ distance means reduced excitability and vice versa. The firing rate of the neuron depends on T/σ through the Gaussian probability distribution function. Specifically, at low firing rate:

$$\text{Firing rate} \simeq K. \frac{1}{\sqrt{2\pi}} \frac{}{T/\sigma} \int^{\infty} e^{-y^2} dy \qquad (1)$$

The integral on the right-hand side gives the probability that the trans-membrane potential will be above threshold. The constant K used to translate this probability into firing rate depends on the frequency content of the membrane potential fluctuations and on the refractory periods of the cell. Its value should be somewhere between 150 and 1000. One thousand is used throughout this representation as the value for K. This value will give the upper bound of T/σ values.

3.4 Sources of Excitatory Inputs

In the previous sections we saw that the ongoing activity of the cortical nerve cells is fairly close to a random Poisson process, that there are good reasons to believe that synaptic activity from all parts of the dendritic tree affects the firing of the cell, and that the magnitude of the transmembrane potential fluctuations determines the firing rate of neurons. In this section we attempt to combine all these points to build a simple model of how the neurons in a network excite each other and so generate a steady firing level.

In the following, the assumptions and the conclusions of the model are spelled out in detail, while the mathematical derivations which are not necessary to understand the conclusions are omitted. A detailed description of this model may be found in Abeles (1981).

a) Assumptions

1. Each neuron in the network accepts contacts from N neurons (and makes contacts with N neurons). These contacts are either excitatory or inhibitory in unknown proportion.

2. Each excitatory postsynaptic potential looks like a falling exponential $A \cdot \exp(-t/\tau)$. Each inhibitory postsynaptic potential looks like: $-A \cdot \exp -A \cdot \exp(-t/\tau)$. Figure 6C shows the hypothetical shape of these potentials. All the synaptic potentials are of equal amplitude (A) and time constant (τ).

3. All the nerve cells fire at an average rate of λ spikes per second.

4. The different nerve cells have uncorrelated activity.

5. All synaptic potentials sum up in a linear fashion.

These assumptions are zero-order approximation to the real situation, in which different synaptic potentials have different amplitudes and time course, different cells fire at different rates and synaptic potentials interact along a dendritic trunk in a nonlinear fashion (Rall 1967). Nevertheless, this crude model shows that although the individual synapse is quite ineffective, it takes only a few simulteneous EPSP's to make the neuron fire. The exact figures will change somewhat by refining the model, but these results will still hold true in essence.

b) Conclusions

Each post synaptic potential contributes variance of $A^2 \tau/2$. In one second we add up $N \cdot \lambda$ such independent processes and, therefore, the total variance of the intracellular potential is

$$\sigma^2 = N \cdot \lambda \cdot A^2 \tau/2 \tag{2}$$

or

$$\sigma/A = [N\lambda \, \tau/2]^{1/2} \tag{3}$$

Resonable figures for the parameters in Eq. (3) are as follows:
N — the number of cells making synaptic contacts with any given neuron is about 20,000 (Cragg 1975).
λ — the rate of firing of each cell is 5 spikes per second.
τ — the time constant of the post synaptic potential is 2.5×10^{-3} seconds.
Putting these values into Eq. (3) we obtain

$$\sigma/A = [125]^{1/2} \simeq 11 \tag{4}$$

This means that despite the multitude of synaptic potentials which give rise to the fluctuating transmembrane potential, its variation is such that the standard deviation is only 11 times bigger than the average amplitude of the EPSP. Equation (3) shows that this σ/A ratio is proportional to the square root of the parameters N, λ and τ making it relatively insensitive to changes in the values assumed. For instance, if only 5000 independent presynaptic cells (instead of 20,000) converge on a post synaptic cell, the standard deviation of the transmembrane fluctuations will be only 5.5 (instead of 11) times larger than the amplitude of the single EPSP. If the time constant of each postsynaptic potential is 10 ms (instead of 2.5), the standard deviation of the transmembrane fluctuation will be 22 (instead of 11) times bigger than the amplitude of the single EPSP.

In the previous section we showed that the distance of threshold from mean membrane potential T/σ for a nerve cell firing at 5 per second is 2.58 (for K = 1000), thus the ratio of threshold to EPSP amplitude T/A is given by:

$$T/A = T/\sigma \times \sigma/A = 2.58 \times 11 = 29 \tag{5}$$

This means that although tens of thousands of EPSP's converge on the cell every second, each individual EPSP is so big (on the average) that it takes as little as 29 simultaneous EPSP's to get from the average membrane potential to threshold. Both estimates of T/σ and of σ/A are not very sensitive to the values chosen for the parameters K, N, λ, τ, so that within the reasonable physiological limits the ratio between threshold and a single EPSP would not exceed the limits of 10-60.

When we think that 20,000 neurons generate about 100,000 spikes every second, and that all these spikes impinge on a single post-synaptic cell, we expect the amplitude of the post-synaptic potential generated by a single presynaptic spike to be very small. Contrary to this intuitive expectation, the above presentation indicates that the effect of a single pre-synaptic neuron is strong. Only 29 presynaptic spikes will bring the transmembrane potential to threshold. This type of strength is limited, however, to effects that are elicited by synchronous activation of several synapses. The effect of the single synapse is quite poor. At the peak of the EPSP the T/σ distance is reduced from 2.58 to 2.58-2.58/29 = 2.49 and the firing rate of the cell will increase from 5 per second to 6.4 per second, and then decrease with a roughly exponential form back to 5 per second, as shown in Fig. 6D. The total effect of the single EPSP will be to add 0.003 spikes to the postsynaptic neuron. This sort of difference between the low efficiency of asynchroneous integration of many synaptic effects and the strenght of excitation produced by coinciding activity of few cells will be discussed again in Chapter 7.

4 Interactions Between Pairs of Cells

4.1 Cross-Renewal Density

In our studies we recorded in most cases from more than one cell. When a pair of cells was studied we could ask to what extent does the firing of one cell affect that of the other? This question is studied very much after the fashion of studies of responses of cells to stimuli. In the case of stimulus presentation we plot the Peri Stimulus Time Histogram (PSTH) which shows us how the firing rate of the cell depends on the presence of stimulus. In the case of simultaneous recording from two cells we plot the cross-renewal density function, which is computed exactly like the PSTH, but the spikes of one of the cells are used to reset the starting point instead of the stimulus. The results of such computation are plotted in Fig. 7.

The abscissa gives the time that passed from the firing of one cell; the ordinate gives the firing rate of the other cell as a function of that time. In Fig. 7A we see that the firing rate of the second cell fluctuates around its mean and is unaffected by the time of firing of the first cell. As in the case of auto-renewal density, the limited duration of the measurement and the random nature of the cell firing make it difficult to obtain absolutely flat curves. The level within which 99% of the curve should be contained if the two units were firing in an independent Poisson fashion is also plotted.

Whenever one cell excites another we expect to see that after a short delay the rate of firing of the other cell will increase and then fall back to zero. Figure 7B illustrates such relation and Fig. 7C illustrates another case of this sort on an expanded scale. The firing rate of the cell has a time course similar to an intracellular EPSP.

The method of constructing the cross-renewal density is essentially a correlation method in which we correlate the appearance of a spike in one neuron with the appearance of a spike in another. This type of study cannot prove any causal relation between the two events. Nevertheless, we tend to interpret the curves as showing causal relations whenever we know of the existence of (causal) neurophysiological mechanisms that could produce such a curve. Curves such as those in Fig. 7B and C are treated here as if they indeed result from a simple synaptic relation between the cells.

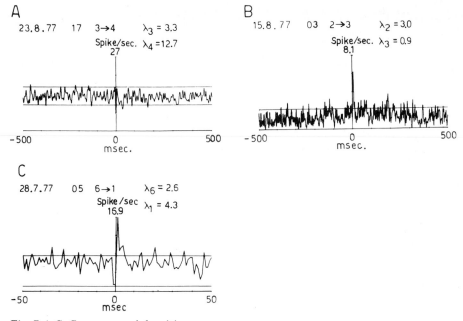

Fig. 7 A-C. Cross renewal densities
The rate of firing of one neuron is shown as a function of time around the firing of another neuron. **A** The two neurons fire independently. **B** One neuron fires at higher rate
for a short time after the other neuron fired. **C** As in **B** but on expanded time scale

4.2 Types of Cross-Renewal Densities

The most abundant cross-renewal seen in the unanethetized, muscle re-
laxed cat is the flat curve (Fig. 7A). This type of curve was seen in 45% of
the neuron pairs studied. In the visual cortex of the behaving cat Burns and
Webb (1979) reported that all the pairs show such flat curves.

The second type seen is shown in Fig. 8A and B. There is a peak or a
trough in the cross-renewal density that extends to both sides of the zero
time delay. Let us discuss first the shape as seen in Fig. 8A. There we see
that cell 2 was more likely to fire either a little before of a little after cell
1 fired. That means that cell 1 was also more likely to fire either a little
before or a little after cell 2. (Our methods fail to detect both spikes when
they fire almost simultaneously, see Chapter 2. Therefore, we are unable
to measure the likelihood of both cells firing exactly together). There seem
to exist two simple explanations for this type of curve: (a) cell 1 excited
cell 2 and cell 2 excited cell 1 (reciprocal excitation). (b) both cells 1 and
2 were excited from a common source (common input). Such excitatory
common input increases simultaneously the firing rate of both cells 1 and 2

28.7.77   05

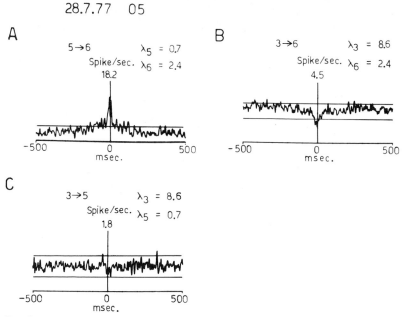

Fig. 8 A-C. Relations among three neurons.
Three single units were recorded simultaneously through the same electrode. All possible relations between pairs are shown. **A** Neurons 1 and 2 share a common input which excites (or inhibits) both of them. **B** Neurons 2 and 3 share a common input which excites one of them and inhibits the other. **C** Neurons 1 and 3 fire independently

during that increased excitability period sometimes cell 1 fired first and sometimes cell 2. The resulting renewal density should show a bilateral peak.

Of the two alternatives, reciprocal excitation and common input, the latter hypothesis is more attractive. The likelihood of two cells exciting each other reciprocally is low, and the time course of the slopes of the peaks of Fig. 8A is too long. Furthermore, in the visual cortex of the cat, the cross-renewal density of most pairs switched from a flat curve into a curve with a peak around zero delay when the cat went to sleep (Burns and Webb 1979). Such changes of shape are readily interpreted by assuming that the appearance of a peak during sleep is brought about by the synchronizing influences of subcortical nuclei. Here we shall treat all cross-renewal density curves with bilateral peak as resulting from a common input driving both cells.

Although the description above was given for an excitatory common input, it holds true also for a common input inhibiting both cells, though there the slopes of the peak are likely to be shallower.

Twenty eight percent of the pairs show such signs of common input. This figures may be appropriate only for the type of preparation that we used (unanesthetized, muscle-relaxed cat) because common inputs may disappear and reappear as the animal changes its arousal state. As explained above, we are unable to tell in which cases the common input is excitatory and in which cases it is inhibitory.

Bilateral troughs such as in Fig. 8B are seen in only 2% of the pairs. These troughs again may be the result of two processes: (a) cell 1 inhibits cell 2 and cell 2 inhibits cell 1 (mutual inhibition), or (b) The two cells are driven by a common source which excites one of them and inhibits the other (common input with opposite effects). Again, the second mechanism, based on common input, is more probable.

The cross-renewal density indicating an excitatory synapse was already discussed (Fig. 7B and C). This type of relation was found only in 12.5% of the pairs. In 8 % of the pairs we saw a transient decrease of the firing rate of one cell following the firing of the other cell. These are interpreted as indicating a connection through an inhibitory synapse between the two cells.

The rest of the pairs (4.5%) showed irregular cross-renewal that could not be reproduced or classified in any simple way.

4.3 Synaptic Relations Between Adjacent Neurons

In the previous chapter we tried to build a model of a network of corti-cal neurons exciting each other in some random fashion. We arrived at the conclusion that a single contact between neurons appears to be inefficient when the number of postsynaptic spikes elicited by each presynaptic spike is considered (0.003). The contact between two cells appears to be quite strong when amplitude of the EPSP relative to threshold (T/A) ratio is considered (29). Can we corroborate these conclusions from the more di-rect measurements of the cross-renewal density?

Let us examine again the peak representing an EPSP as seen in the cross-renewal density of Fig. 7C. The area under the peak is 0.05 spikes. Thus, each spike of cell 1 elicits on the average 0.05 spikes in cell 2. The rate of firing of cell 2 is increased from its ongoing spontaneous rate of 2.6 per sec-ond to 10 per second at the peak of the EPSP. From these figures, using Eq. (1), we compute the distance of threshold from resting potential (T/σ) to be 2.8 during spontaneous activity and 2.33 at the peak of the EPSP. The difference between these two T/σ distances is the amplitude of the EPSP expressed in A/σ. From all these we may compute the T/A ratio, that is how many such EPSP's are required to get to threshold. In the case of the synaptic contact responsible for Fig. 7C we obtain T/A = 6.

On the average in all the synaptic contacts seen by us the area under the hill representing the EPSP was 0.06 spikes and the average ratio T/A was

7.7. Although these figures are considerably higher than the 0.003 spikes and 29 computed for the average synapse in the previous chapter, the two main points of the calculations of synaptic strength in the previous chapter are corroborated:

a) Contact between two cells seems weak when we ask the question: How many spikes does each presynaptic spike elicit?

b) Contact between two cells seems strong when we ask the question: How many such EPSP's have to be added synchronously to reach threshold?

The discrepancy between the strength of our measured synaptic effects and the calculated average synapse is attributed to two factors. We measure from two cells whose somata are close together; contacts between such cells are expected to be stronger than the average contact. The statistical nature of our estimate of cross-renewal density is such that we can easily detect strong effects while we never collected enough data to able to detect weak effects. Hence, our sampling is biased toward pairs of cells with strong synaptic contacts.

To summarize: the computed average synaptic effect described in the previous chapter is weaker than the measured synaptic effect between adjacent neurons, but has essentially the same features as revealed by the cross-renewal density between the neurons.

Most physiologists agree that the activity of cortical neurons is held down by strong inhibitory effects. This view is supported both by theoretical considerations (e.g., Beurle 1956) which indicate that without inhibitory feedback cortical activity would either fade out or build to epileptic seizure, by intracellular recording from cortical neurons (e.g., de Ribaupierre and Goldstein 1972), and by intracortical stimulation (Hess et al. 1975). In our studies only 8% of the pairs showed inhibitory relations. Although this figure seems low, it has to be compared with the 12% of pairs showing excitatory synaptic relations. If both figures represent truly the connectivity of the cortical network then 40% of the intracortical synapses are inhibitory while 60% of the intracortical synapses are excitatory. This is a high proportion when compared with anatomical estimates of intracortical inhibition.

It is thought that the intracortical inhibition is generated by stellate cells. Although it is not known absolutely that all the pyramidal cells are excitatory and all the stellate cells are inhibitory, the proportion of stellate cells to pyramidal cells may be used to obtain an order of magnitude estimate for the intracortical inhibition. In the visual cortex of the cat, Sholl (1956) found that 20% of the neurons are stellate cells while 80% are pyramidal, while Mitra (1955) found for both visual and somato sensory cortices of the cat a ratio of stellates to pyramidal cells of 35/63.

Another way by which excitatory synapses may be differentiated from inhibitory ones is by their morphology. On several occasions where electrophysiological measurements indicated the existence of inhibitory synapses it was possible to identify the synapses by electron microscopy as having flat vesicles and symmetrical membrane thickening, while excitatory synapses had round vesicles and asymmetrical membrane thickening. Although it is not clear that these differences are accurate also for the cortex, the proportion of symmetrical synapses to asymmetrical synapses may be used to obtain an order of magnitude estimate for the intracortical inhibition. Fisken et al. (1975) made small lesions in the visual cortex of monkeys and then counted the number of degenerating synapses of the two types at various distances from the lesion. They found that only 9% of the synapses were of symmetrical type. Mather et al. (1978) found that 37% of the synapses in the visual cortex of the rabbit had flatened vesicles.

In view of the anatomical evidence, our direct measurement in which 40% of the contacts between neighbors are inhibitory is certainly not on the low side. What seems low is that only 8% of the pairs studied showed such contacts. This issue will be discussed again in Section 4.5.

4.4 Sources of Excitation Within Groups of Neurons

The calculation of mean synaptic strength made in Chapter 3 was based on the assumption that many inputs converge on each cell and that their activity is independent. Do these assumptions still hold when interactions between two units are studied?

The independence between firing patterns of different neurons is only partially correct. About half the pairs studied had flat cross-renewal density and are, therefore, completely independent, but in about 30% we had common inputs and their activity is partially synchronized. How strong is this synchronization? One way to estimate its strength is by converting the cross-renewal density into correlation coefficients, which is done by the formula

$$\rho = \Delta T(\lambda_1 \lambda_{2/1} - \lambda_1 \lambda_2)/[(\lambda_1 - \lambda_1^2 \Delta T)/(\lambda_2 - \lambda_2^2 \Delta T)]^{1/2}$$

where ρ is the correlation coefficient λ_1 and λ_2 are the average rates of firing of the two cells, $\lambda_{2/1}$ is the peak value of the cross-renewal density between cell 2 and cell 1, and ΔT is the width of the bin used to compute the cross-renewal density. Using bins of 5 ms, which are of the order of magnitude of the EPSP, we obtain for the common input of Fig. 8A $\rho = 0.026$. The average correlation coefficient in our data was $\rho = 0.06$. Thus, although the common inputs have a clear effect on the firing rate of the cells as seen in the cross-renewal density, this effect represents only feeble correlation between the firing of the neurons.

The assumption of independence is therefore fairly accurate. The multiplicity of sources of excitation and inhibition impinging on every cell is clearly indicated by the anatomy of the cortex but has been difficult to demonstrate physiologically.

Most single-unit studies were made in sensory areas and there the columnar organization and the mapping of the sensory periphery are thought to indicate that large numbers of neurons are controlled by the same sensory inputs. The spontaneous activity of units is thought to be under strong control of the reticular formation and its continuation in the diffuse thalamic projection system. These concepts may be taken as indicating a situation where only few incoming fibers control many of the cortical neurons within a column, but our studies of the auditory cortex indicate that this is not the case. Let us first examine the common inputs within a small group of neurons.

Occasionally we see several pairs with signs of common inputs among units recorded simultaneously at the same spot. In such cases we can ask whether the correlations are due to one and the same source, or whether they represent independent sources. In Fig. 8 we see a simple example for this type of analysis. We recorded from three units simultaneously and could, therefore, study the cross-renewal density for three pairs of units. Cells 1 and 2 showed signs of common input with similar effects on both units. Cells 2 and 3 showed signs of common input with antagonistic effects (Fig. 8B). If all these effects were due to a single common source which drives this group of three neurons we can make the following prediction: cells 1 and 2 fire in phase while cells 2 and 3 fire in antiphase therefore cells 3 and 1 should also fire in antiphase. Then, we would expect to find that the cross-renewal between cells 3 and 1 will show signs of common inputs with antagonistic effects. The flat cross-renewal density between cells 3 and 1 (Fig. 8C) forces us to conclude that the source of common input to cells 1 and 2 is different and independent of the source of common input to cells 2 and 3.

In one case, while recording from six cells simultaneously, we found that five of the cells were affected by such common inputs. Within these five cells we could construct ten pairs, all of which showed common inputs; however, by comparing with other units and by studies of three-cell correlations (see Chap. 6) we could show that these represent ten different sources of common inputs with uncorrelated activity. It is difficult to find one common source that affects more than two cells. In fact we had only one case where the same common input affected three cells, and even then the effect was weak.

In summary we can detect within a small group of neurons the effect of several (up to 10) sources of input which act independently. The limitations of our method do not allow us to demonstrate the thousands of inputs which are known to exist anatomically, because we can detect a source of inputs only when it affects two cells from the group of cells under study, while independence between sources can be demonstrated only when two pairs of cells are affected by such common inputs. Nevertheless, our finding that almost always all the inputs that can be detected are independent indicates that the thousands of other inputs (which cannot be demonstrated by our method) also act independently.

The sources discussed so far are active when no external auditory stimulus is present. What about sensory inputs to the cortex? This question will be dealt in detail in Chapter 5, in which we show that the sensory input to a group of neurons is composed also of several independent sources.

4.5 Is the Cortical Network Randomly Connected?

The representation of data so far gives the impression that we face a network of cells whose connectivity is controlled by chance only. We want here to reexamine this question more closely from two points of view.

a) are there cell specializations?

b) are the connectivity figures obtained by the different methods consistent?

One could imagine that some cells in the cortex specialize in distributing their synapses to adjacent neurons, while others send their axon some distance away before starting to give synapses. In this case when we record from a group of neurons and find that one of the cells makes a synaptic contact with its neighbor we would expect it also to make synaptic contacts with the other neighbors — or at least we would expect it to have higher probability of making synaptic contact with the other neighbors. This kind of organization might be true for excitatory contacts, inhibitory contacts, or both.

Another possible arrangement could be of cells specializing in receiving information from their adjacent neighbors. In this case, if a cell within a group is found to receive a synapse from one of the members of the group it should be more likely that it receives also synaptic contacts from other members of the group. Again, it is possible that such receptive cells exist only for inhibitory synapses, only for excitatory synapses or for both types.

Statistical analysis of the distribution of such cells within the groups did not reveal any significant deviation from chance. Thus, in this respect the network of local connection seems random. However, the small number of cells from which we could record simultaneously (3-6) and the inability of our methods to detect weak interactions between neurons make it impossible to be absolutely sure about the randomness of the connections. All that can be said is that deviations from complete chance, if they exist at all, are not very strong.

We did find a strong tendency of common inputs to be distributed unevenly among groups. In some groups almost all the pairs showed independent activity while in others many pairs seem to have common inputs. One has to bear in mind that common input may appear or disappear as the animal goes to sleep or wakes up. Since the state of wakefulness was not systematically controlled, it is not clear whether this uneven distribution of common inputs reflects functional differences among the groups of neurons, or is it just a reflection of the different arousal states of our experimental animals.

We can now compare, on a quantitative basis, the measured interactions between neurons with the interactions calculated when a random network of chance connections is assumed. This comparison will qualify somewhat our connectivity figures and show the kind of problems encountered when cortical connectivity is studied quantitatively. If the reader is not interested in this statistical approach he may skip the rest of this chapter.

We shall base our estimates of interaction strength and abundance on two sets of connectivity figures:

a) The probability and strength of connections as calculated by the measurements of cross-renewal densities between pairs of cells in the auditory cortex of the unanesthetized, muscle-relaxed cat.

b) The probability and strength of connections as evaluated from anatomy and from the model of superposition of synaptic potentials described in the previous chapter.

Let P be the probability of a given neuron to make synaptic contact with another given neuron. Then when we measure activity of two cells we have a probability of $2P-P^2$ of observing a contact between the two cells, because either one cell contacts the other (probability P) or the other cell contacts the first cell (probability P) or both cells contact each other (probability P^2).

In our data we found in 12% of the cross-renewal densities signs of excitatory relations and in 8% signs of inhibitory relations (Chap. 1 and 2). This means that the probability of excitatory contact between two cells was about 0.06 and of inhibitory contact about 0.04. The strength of the contacts (measured as explained in Chap. 4.3) was such that each presynaptic spike adds (or deletes) 0.06 spikes to the spike train of the postsynaptic cell. This set of figures will be referred to as the measured connectivity.

The anatomical connectivity in the cat's cortex will be derived after the fashion introduced by Braitenberg (1981) for the mouse. Let us examine a typical cortical neuron and evaluate the synaptic contacts it makes with its neighbors. The axon of this neuron branches locally and extends on the average a quarter of mm away on each side of the main shaft. The branches might be distributed within a cube of 0.5 x 0.5 x 0.5 mm, having within this region a total length of 8 mm. The axon gives off a synapse about every micron so that is makes 8000 synapses. We assume that these synapses are made at random (which implies that they are made essentially with different neurons) so that our neuron contacts locally 8000 other neurons whose somata are contained within the cube described above but also some distance away (Fig. 9). Since the dendrites of the receptive neurons may spread as far as a quarter of a millimeter on each side of the cell body (we do not consider here the apical branching of the pyramidal cell), the cell bodies of two neurons may be as far as half a millimeter away from each other and can still make direct contact (see also Braitenberg 1978a, b). In this way a neuron may contact other neurons whose cell bodies lie within a 1 x 1 x 1 mm cube. This volume contains in the cat about 40,000 cells, of which 8000 are contacted by our neuron. Therefore, the probability of contact between two neurons is 8000/40000 = 0.2.

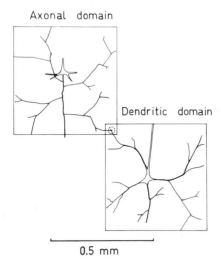

Fig. 9. Axonal and dendritic domains of cortical neurons.
The intracortical axonal collaterals are assumed to branch within 0.5 x 0.5 x 0.5 mm cube and so do the dendrites. The maximal distance between the cell bodies of neurons that contact each other is 0.5 mm. The drawing of neurons is schematic, the size of the cell body, the thickness of axons and of dendrites is exaggerated

Some of the neurons make excitatory contacts and some make inhibitory contacts. On the basis of our cross-renewal studies we assume a ratio of 0.6 excitatory to 0.4 inhibitory contacts. The strength of contacts will be assumed to be 0.003 as calculated in Chapter 3.4, where the ongoing activity of the single neuron was analyzed. That is, we assume that each presynaptic spike when added to the ongoing activity will add (or delete) on the average 0.003 spikes to the spike train of the postsynaptic cell. This set of figures will be referred to as the *anatomical connectivity*.

The values obtained from the anatomical connectivity differ from the measured ones. Anatomically, the probability of synaptic contact between two cells is twice as large; the strength of the average contact is 20-fold weaker. This discrepancy is partly because of the bias of the methods of measurement, namely, the neurons from which the measured data were derived are always close neighbors and therefore do not represent a fair sample of all neurons that make synaptic contacts; in addition the cross-renewal analysis is not sentitive to weak synaptic interactions. These limitations bias our sample toward the stronger synapses and may account, at least in part, for both the lower probability and the higher strength of the measured synapses.

The discrepancy between anatomical and measured connectivities may indicate, however, that the anatomical model in which a neuron can affect its neighbors evenly in all directions is an over-simplified one. This possibility will be reexamined in the next chapter. Here we turn now to examine our data further by comparing the measured strength and abundance of common inputs with what may be expected anatomically.

The expected number of pairs with common inputs may be calculated in the following way. Around the first neuron in each pair there are about 8000 cells that affect its activity. Of these, on the average 8000 x 0.2 cells will contact also the other neuron in the pair. Thus, for each pair there should be about 1600 sources of common inputs in the nearby vicinity. The effects of such sources are, however, very weak. The probability that a spike of such common source will fire both neurons in synchrony is on the average 0.003 x 0.003 = 0.000009. All of the 1600 sources of common input, each of which fires at 5 per second, add up to 5 x 1600 x 0.003 x 0.003 = 0.072, occurrences of spikes in both units of the pairs per second. This is probably too weak to be detected by our methods. But these calculated figures are just the expected average. In some cases the pair may have less than 1600 sources of common input and in some more. In some cases the effects of the common inputs will be weaker and in some stronger. Therefore, it is possible that in some cases the effect of common inputs will be strong enough to generate a significant peak in the cross-renewal density curves. It is not clear whether the anatomical connectivity can justify the 30% of pairs with the observed strength of common inputs. One would need a quantitative model, taking into account also the scatter of connectivity and synaptic strength, in order to test the agreement between the anatomical and measured estimates of the abundance and strength of the common inputs. It is likely that such a model would lead to the conclusion that the observed common inputs are not derived from the local intracortical network, but are brought into the cortex from other places (such as thalamus or reticular formation) and are governed by other laws of connectivity.

Can we obtain reasonable estimates when basing our calculations on the measured connectivity? There we set the probability of one cell giving a synapse to the other at 0.1. If we assume again that this connectivity is true for 40,000 cells around the measured neuron we have 4000 cells connected to one member of the pair. Of these, there should be 4000 x 0.1 = 400 cells that connect also to the other − this is fourfold less than estimated from the anatomical data, but the measured synaptic strength is much bigger − being 0.06 postsynaptic spikes per presynaptic spike. According to this figure we should have per presynaptic spike on the average 0.06 x 0.06 = 0.0036 cases where both cells in the pair fire synchronously. The effect of all the 400 common inputs, each of which fires at 5 per second, on the pair would combine to 5 x 400 x 0.06 x 0.06 = 7.2, which is easily detectable by our methods. This means that if all the units within 1 mm^3 were connected as measured in our experiments we expect to find a common input for every pair studied. This is not the case either in our experiments nor in those of Burns and Webb (1979). The simplest conclusions is that the strong synapses measured by us are not distributed throughout the volume of 1 mm^3 but exist only between close neighbors. If we limit the volume through which these strong synapses are distributed to 0.4 x 0.4 x 0.4 mm^3 we come to the range of reasonable agreement between the measured number of pairs with common inputs and the calculated number.

The assumptions made in these calculations are very crude; we did not take into account the distribution of firing rates among neurons, the distribution of large and small dendritic domains and of axonal domains or the direction of spread of axon collaterals relative to the soma. At the present stage the low sensitivity of the analysis cannot support a more refined model, but it points to a direction which quantitative analysis of cortical connectivity can take.

In summary our data support the view that each cortical cell receives and makes many local connections. They indicate that neurons in close proximity can make strong contacts, while remote neurons make weaker contacts. They show clearly that most pairs of cells show independent of slightly correlated activity. There is nothing in the data to indicate any distinct classes of units with very specialized types of connectivity, but the possibility that different cell kinds tend to have different patterns of connectivity in a statistical sense cannot be excluded.

5 Responses to Sound

The response properties of sensory areas are thought by many neuro-physiologists to be arranged neatly along maps (somatotopic, retinotopic, and tonotopic maps) and parcelled into columns within which all units share some common properties. There have been two approaches to this organization. In one, the order of the arrangement is stressed (e.g., Hubel and Wiesel 1979, Mountcastle 1979) while the other approach stresses the statistical nature of the arrangement (e.g., Creuzfeldt 1978, Towe 1975). The debate between these approaches has been especially prolonged in the case of the auditory cortex because its organization has resisted the experimental approaches for detection of order more than the somatosensory or visual areas. The reader is referred to Merzenich et al. (1975), Imig and Adrian (1977), and Middlebrooks et al. (1980) for examples of work stressing the order in the cortex and to Evans et al. (1965), Abeles and Goldstein (1970), Goldstein and Abeles (1975) for works stressing the statistical nature of the order. These global properties of the arrangement of the auditory cortex are related to our study of local cortical circuits only indirectly. If the tonotopic mapping of the auditory cortex is very strict, we expect that when measuring the activity of a group of cells, all the cells would respond to tones of similar pitch. If the columnar parcellation of the auditory cortex is very strict, we expect to find strong correlations between neighbors when a stimulus is applied. These arguments may lead one to believe that when we record from a group of neurons while applying an adequate stimulus the whole group would respond in unison.

5.1 Stating the Problem

Let us consider the following hypothetical problem. If we could find a stimulus that excites most of the neurons within a small cortical column (say 0.25 x 0.25 x 2 mm) we would face the following situation: This column contains some 5000 neurons. If most of them are excited together they are going to convey a lot of synaptic excitation to their immediate neighbors. Each neighbor will receive about 0.06 x 5000 = 300 excitatory inputs during a short period, which is much more than required to make it fire. Hence, at the next stage all the neighboring cells will fire too, and they in turn will excite their neighbors and so on.

Such a spread of transcortical excitation is seen when epileptic seizures spread through the cortex but they do not exist in response to any natural stimulus. Two possible mechanisms to prevent this spread may be considered (a) sensory stimuli that excite one region of the cortex also generate a surround inhibition that prevents the spread of the excitation laterally; (b) sensory stimuli do not strongly excite large groups of cells in one region.

In the next section we shall see that a group of neurons generally would not respond in unison.

5.2 Responses of Groups of Neurons to Sound

In a series of experiments Ron Frostig studied responses of groups of neurons to sound. Recordings were made from the auditory cortex of unanesthetized but muscle-relaxed cats. The stimuli were always delivered in the following schedule: 1 s of silence was followed by 8 s of stimulation with tone, band pass noise or wide band noise and then again there was 1 s of silence. Two forms of stimuli were mainly used. A frequency sweep in which the pitch of the sound was changed from 100 Hz to 20 kHz in 4 s and then back to 100 Hz in 4 s. This kind of stimulus scans the frequency range so that the responses of the unit to a wide range of frequencies may be seen. The frequency was changed exponentially with time and in addition the tone was turned on and off every 10 ms. In the second form the frequency of the stimulus was constant. The tone was turned on for 0.1 s followed by 0.9 s of silence; this type of stimulus was repeated many times to allow for quantitative plotting of the response by measuring the firing rate of the units as a function of time. In Fig. 10 we see an example of the responses of six single units to a frequency sweep.

Responses of each unit are plotted in a separate strip. Time is plotted on the abscissa. First we see the activity of the unit during 1 s of silence, then, at the vertical line, the 100 Hz tone starts and goes up to 20 kHz within 4 s. Throughout this period whenever a spike is fired we plot a dot at the appropriate time. After reaching 20 kHz the frequency sweeps back to 100 Hz and the firing of the unit is represented by dots on the upper band. At the end of the down-going sweep we see again the activity during 1 s of silence. This whole process is repeated 12 times and for each repetition the dots are plotted a little higher than for the previous line. In this way we have for each unit two bands of dots. In the lower band we see the respon-

23.8.77   15

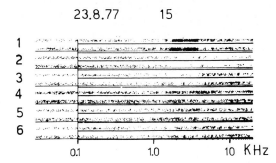

Fig. 10. Response of six units to tone sweeps.
The *six strips* show the responses of six single units to tones swept from 100 Hz to 20 kHz exponentially. Within each strip the *lower band* shows the responses to an up-going sweep and the *upper band* to down-going sweep. (By courtesy of R. Frostig)

ses to the up-going sweep, while in the upper band we see the response to the down-going sweep.

In Fig. 10 we see that unit 1 responded very strongly to frequencies between 1.7 and 4 kHz both on the up- and down-going sweep. Unit 3 showed some suppression in the frequencies of band 1.7-4 kHz, but had an excitatory response at a higher frequency range (5-14 kHz), while unit 3 showed some suppression in both the lower and higher frequency bands. Units 4, 5, and 6 do not seem to respond to any of the stimuli.

Two points are evident: (a) The group of units studied do show some preference to certain frequencies; (b) There is no single frequency that would make all the units (or even a considerable fraction of the units) fire together.

Figure 11 illustrates other examples for the responses of several units to sweeps. Within each group one can observe some units that respond to common frequency range, but other units having a different response range and units with no clear response could also be observed. Thus, although the response properties are not distributes in a completely random fashion, there is also no one appropriate stimulus that would make the entire group fire vigorously. This type of probabilistic organization of response within the group was found for all the cases studied.

When the stimuli were limited to a narrow frequency range we could repeat them many times and detect even very weak responses. Figure 12 shows the responses of the same units as in Fig. 10 to tone peeps around 2.5 kHz presented once per second. Again unit 1 shows a clear excitatory response, while unit 2 shows some suppression. When responses to several hundreds of stimuli are averaged and plotted as PSTH (Fig. 13) it seems that the 2.5 kHz affects all the units.

If we wished to stress the uniformity within the groups we could say that for almost all the recording sites we could find at least one type of stimulus that would affect the firing of all the cells. If we wished to stress the diversity we could say that in no recording site could we find a stimu-

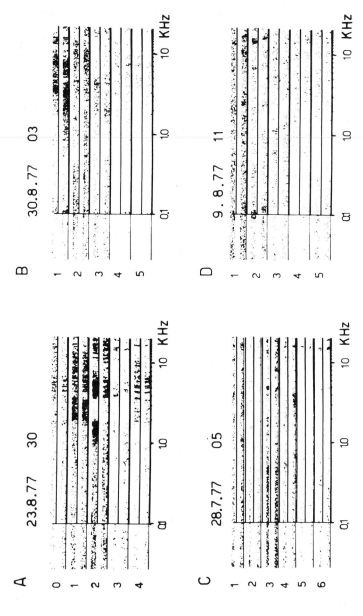

Fig. 11. Response of groups of units to tone sweeps.
Responses of few groups of cells from different experiments are shown. Same representation as in Fig. 10.
(By courtesy of R. Frostig)

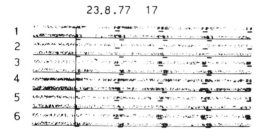

23.8.77   17

Fig. 12. Responses of six units to tones around 2.5 kHz.
The unit responses are plotted as in Fig. 10, but the tones are turned on only during the time underlined by the *small bar*. The frequency of the tones changes only little from one tone to another so that all the responses might be considered as coming from one frequency range. (By courtesy of R. Frostig)

23.8.77   17 02

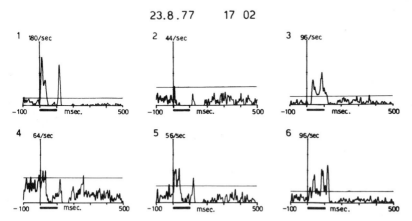

Fig. 13. Responses of 6 units to tones around 2.5 kHz.
The data of Fig. 12 is presented as PSTH where the rate of firing is plotted against time. All units responded to this tone but some of the responses are weak. The different units show a variety of response patterns. (By courtesy of R. Frostig)

lus that would strongly excite most of the cells in the group, but at every site we could find different stimuli that strongly excite different cells.

The same picture was found when two types of band pass noise instead of pure tones were used, and when recording the responses of groups of cells to tone or to band pass noise sweeps in the auditory cortex of behaving monkeys.

In summary: when a group of nerve cells is activated by an external stimulus it would not respond in unison. Here too, as in the spontaneous activity, we find multiple sensory inputs driving the units in the group. This multiplicity of sources of information is evident also when the patterns of responses are considered. There was no tendency of the groups of neurons to share a common response pattern. However, this does not mean that the connections are completely random. Rather, at every point we see that some frequency ranges are more effective than others so there are definitely some statistical rules about connectivity of the incoming information from the thalamus to the cortex (see Frostig et al. 1982 for more details about these experiments). Coming back to our problem, there is no danger that an appropriate stimulus will trigger an epileptic fit because no such stimulus excites simultaneously a whole column of units in the cortex. The diversity of response ranges and firing patterns in a group of neurons suggests that some complex processing could be carried out by the cortical network. This possibility is investigated further in the next two sections.

5.3 Stability of the Cortical Network

In the previous chapter we saw that for some pairs of units we could detect signs of common inputs driving both units, for some we could see signs of synaptic interactions, while many others fired independently. Is this picture a stable one, or do the external conditions change it?

To answer this question we want to compare relations between units in two states. For example, when the relations in wakefulness were compared with the relations in sleep, Burns and Webb (1979) found that common source driving both units appears in sleep. In our experiments, R. Frostig studied the effect of presentation of stimuli on the relations between units. In this type of measurement one has first to eliminate the effect of the stimulus itself. Assume for example that a given stimulus excites both cells simultaneously; if we compute the cross-renewal density for the pair while the stimulus is on, we must see a hill around the zero delay time. This hill represents a common input, but it might very well be due to the excitation generated secondarily by the stimulus. Dickson and Gerstein (1974) overcame this problem by the following procedure: For one of the cells they considered the times of firing in relation to one stimulus presentation while the times of firing of the other cell were taken around a different stimulus, and then they computed the cross-renewal density. If all the effects seen were time-locked to the stimulus this shuffling would not affect the shape of the cross-renewal density. On the other hand, if the neurons had some functional relations which are not time-locked to the stimulus the shuffling would wipe them out completely. In the ordinary cross-renewal density we see both the effects of the stimuli on the two units and the effects due to other relations (synaptic coupling or common inputs) between the units. In the cross-renewal density computed after shuffling the times, we see only the effect of the stimulus on the units. If we substract the two graphs from each other we are left with the effects which are not time-locked to the stimuli. The shape of this differential cross-renewal density could then be compared to the cross-renewal density when no stimulus was presented.

Any change in the shape of the cross renewal indicates change in the relations between the units which is due to the presence of stimulus but not time-locked to the stimulus. We see an example of such a change in Fig. 14.

Both cells 1 and 2 responded to stimulation by noise bursts, the cross-renewal density (Fig. 14C) shows indeed that a common input is driving both units. After shuffling the times of stimuli to cell 2 the cross-renewal density (Fig. 14D) still shows the same common input. In the differential renewal density we see only random fluctuations around the zero line. This means that during stimulation the relations between the units were time-locked to the stimulus. This is in contrast to the cross-renewal density obtained between the two units during no stimulation (Fig. 14F). Thus, there is a common input driving the two cells when no stimulus is present, and this common input is replaced by a common input which is locked to the stimulus when a stimulus is presented.

How is this change to be interpreted? Either the sources of common input seen during spontaneous activity are inhibited by the stimulus and at the same time the two cells are excited by other sources which are time-locked to the stimulus (Fig. 14G), or, the same common sources are seen both in the stimulation and the no-stimulation period. However, during stimulation their activity becomes strongly time-locked to the stimulus (Fig. 14H). Such sources of common input may reside in the Medial Geniculate Body (MGB) of the thalamus, from which the sensory information to the auditory cortex is derived, or, if they are in the cortex they are controlled by the activity of neurons in the medial geniculate body.

One third of the common inputs seen during no stimulation disappeared in the differential renewal density for at least one type of stimulus.

Thus, about one third of the input to our neurons is controlled tightly by some auditory stimulus. Where does the rest of the input come from? Anatomically the medial geniculate body is the only place which projects massively into the primary cortex. However, the total number of axons arriving at the auditory cortex is probably much larger than the number of cells in the MGB. The rest of the fibers do not seem to come from any confined region but are derived from very many (perhaps all) cortical areas as well as from other deeper nuclei of the brain. What then is the role of the other two-thirds of inputs? This question will be discussed in Chapter 6.

Here we proceed to discuss the question of stability of synaptic relations. In about 12% of the pairs we observed a cross-renewal density suggesting an excitatory synaptic relation. In 12 out of 15 pairs this synaptic relation was not seen in the differential renewal density for at least one type of stimulus. How could a synapse disappear by stimulation?

There are several ways to account for such a change. In the first place, what may seem a synaptic relation may be a common input displaced to

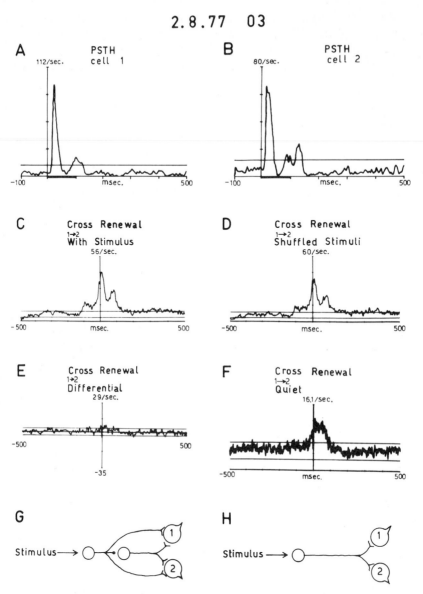

Fig. 14 A-H. Changes in the relations between units during stimulus presentation.
A PSTH for unit #1. **B** PSTH for unit #2. Both **A** and **B** were obtained simultaneously
by stimulating with wide band noise burst. **C** The cross-renewal density between the
units while the stimulus is present. **D** The cross-renewal density after shuffling of stimuli. **E** The differential renewal density (**C** minus **D**) is flat showing that all the effects seen
in **C** are time-locked to the stimulus. **F** The cross-renewal density when no stimulus is
present. **G, H** Two possible mechanisms to explain the difference between **E** and **F**. (By
courtesy of R. Frostig)

one side of the cross-renewal curve. That is a common input with very narrow time course that affects one cell well before it affects the other. An alternative explanation is that the synapse(s) connecting the two cells may be suppressed (by presnypatic inhibition) by the incoming sensory driven activity. This should generally only reduce the effectiveness of the synapse, but with our detection methods such reduction could easily make the signs of synaptic interaction disappear in the noise. In effect any reduction in firing rate of one (or both) units in the studied pair will reduce the chance of detecting a synaptic relation. The last possibility is that what seems a direct synaptic interaction is mediated through interneurons. In this case the interneurons may be inhibited by the incoming sensory activity.

This last explanation seems the simplest and we wish here to explore this possibility quantitatively; such exploration will shed some further light on the connectivity within the cortex.

When we see signs of synaptic interaction after a short delay we assume that this reflects a monosynaptic relation. However, our time resolution (1 ms) is too poor to state with confidence that the relation is mono- bi- or even tri-synaptic. We assume that the weakness of the synapses makes it unlikely to detect any relation between the two cells if more than one synapse had to be traversed. However, there are multiple parallel ways to get from one neuron to another if we allow interneurons to be interposed.

If we use our anatomical connectivity data we obtain the following estimate for the strength of excitatory bisynaptic connection between two cells. A given excitatory neuron is connected to 40,000 x 0.2 = 8000 neurons around it. Of these 8000 neurons, 5600 (8000 x 0.6) are of excitatory type. If we chose another neuron there will be, on the average, 5600 x 0.2 = 1120 interneurons interposed between the two cells. Despite the low probability (0.14) of obtaining a direct excitatory synapse between the two neurons, there are many parallel ways by which excitation from a given neuron can reach another given neuron through one interneuron. This situation is demonstrated on a small group of cells in Fig. 15. Sixteen cells are shown, each cell gives an excitatory synapse to four cells. In this network almost every cell may be affected by cell 1, either directly or through one interneuron. Some cells may be affected by two parallel pathways. Thus, there are two parallel bisynaptic pathways from cell 1 to cell 6 (through cells 3 and 13).

Let us turn back to the cortical network. We found that on the average every two adjacent neurons are connected through 1120 excitatory "interneurons". When one of the cells fires it evokes on the average 0.003 spikes in each of these 1120 interneurons. That is in the whole population 3.36 (1120 x 0.003) spikes are evoked. Each of these evoke again 0.003 spikes in the target neuron; so that their combined effect is 0.01 spikes in the target neuron. When we use the connectivity values obtained from our direct meas-

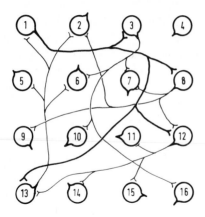

Fig. 15. Schematic representation of a random network.
Only the connections of cell #1 and of the cells contacted by cell #1 are shown. Although cell #1 contacts only a quarter of the cells directly, it can affect almost every cell indirectly. Some cells, such as #6, are affected by cell #1 through *two parallel* pathways

urements (instead of the anatomical connectivity) we obtain similar strength for the excitatory bisynaptic pathways.

Our calculations overestimate the strength in that we did not take into account the presence of inhibitory interneurons, and we also did not take into account the fact that the axonal domain of the interneurons does not necessarily overlap the axonal domain of the first neuron. But even this (over estimated) strength of bisynaptic pathways is too small to be detected by our methods. It is, therefore, not very likely that the synaptic effects we see are mediated through polysynaptic pathways. In Chapter 6, we shall see that when the timing of spikes is not random (but well organized) transmission along polysynaptic pathways may occur.

Let us summarize the results described in this section: We saw that the relations between two units can change with changing conditions. This holds true for common inputs to the pairs as well as for the strength of their synaptic contact. We also found that only about one-third of the inputs to a neuron in the auditory cortex are driven very strongly by sound. All these properties suggest that the cortex is not merely a simple station along the sensory pathway.

5.4 Is the Auditory Cortex a Purely Sensory Station?

One of the common ways to think about sensory systems is to view them as a series of stations; each receives information from the previous one, processes it in some way and sends the results on to the next station. The auditory cortex may also be viewed in this way. Its main input is thought to be from the medial geniculate nucleus of the thalamus and its main output is to the secondary auditory cortices (Pandia et al. 1969, Sousa-Pinto 1973).

This view is often extended to other brain structures and functions. Because of this approach we tend, when we measure single-unit activity during behavior, to give a label to each unit, categorizing it as having a certain function.

As an illustration let us consider an animal that learned to press a lever in response to a certain sound. We think of a sequence of events such as: a stimulus arrives at the sense organ, the information is analyzed stage by stage as it passes through the sensory system, at the end of this analysis certain feature detection neurons are activated. Then these sensory analysers "tell" the animal that this has been the appropriate stimulus and as a result the animal will issue the appropriate response. In Fig. 16 we see a representation of this sequence of events. The stimulus is sorted out by the sensory system and the appropriate stimulus feature is switched to the appropriate motor response by a complex system of the sensory motor association network. There is experimental evidence from animal training experiments indicating that the main thing the animals have to learn is which sensory analyzer is the relevant one in a given situation (Sutherland and Mackintosh 1971).

This form of sequential representation which starts and ends in well-defined anatomical structures often suggests that the other functions are also segregated in well-defined anatomical structures (for instance sensory cortex, association cortex, and motor cortex), or at least that each function has its own group of neurons responsible for its execution.

This hypothesis, that each neuron has only one function, was examined by Eilon Vaadia, in our laboratory. His aim was to create an experimental situation in which one can distinguish among sensory, associative, and motor neuronal activity. Under usual conditions this is impossible, because activities related to each of these processes must take place in the short time lapse between the presentation of the stimulus and emission of the response. Although some segregation in time is expected (sensory activity is likely to be close in time to the stimulus, motor activity is likely to appear just before and during the response, and associative activity is likely to be interposed in between) this segregation cannot be used as a criterion for separating neuronal activity into these three categories.

To overcome these difficulties the following paradigm was devised: A monkey was trained to discriminate between two stimuli, a sine wave (Sa) and a band pass noise (Sb). The monkey was trained to press a lever down in order to initiate one of these two stimuli and then to move the lever to the left when he hears the sine wave (Ra) and to the right when he hears the noise (Rb). This type of stimulus response association is shown in Fig. 17A. When the animal learned this task the required responses were reversed (Fig. 17B), so that in response to Sa he had to make Rb while in response to Sb he had to make Ra. When he learned this task the contin-

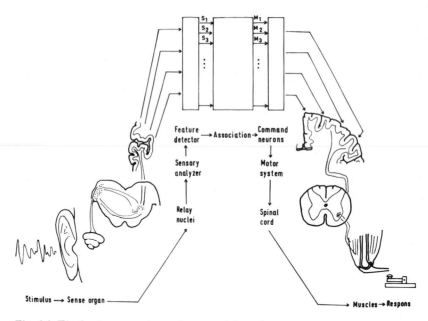

Fig. 16. The brain as a system of sequential stations.
According to this view each neuron and possibly even each brain region plays a role only at one given stage in the sequence of events from stimulus to response

gencies were reversed back to the first ones and so on. After many reversals the monkey would perform along both patterns very well (above 90% success) and switch from one pattern to the other very quickly (within 2 to 20 trials).

At that stage the monkey was anesthetized and prepared for single-unit recordings. After recovery and retraining single units were recorded from its auditory cortex while the monkey performed this discrimination reversal task. Let us see what we expect to record if the brain works along the block diagram of Fig. 16. If we encounter a unit that takes part in the sensory analysis we would expect its activity to depend only on the stimulus used. For instance, it might respond only to Sa and its response will not be affected by the pattern of behavior. That is, we would get the same response if Sa leads to Ra or to Rb. If the unit is part of the motor system its activity should be associated only with the motor response. In contrast to the sensory or motor units an association unit will fire in correlation with

A.   Pattern 0   B.   Pattern 1

    Sa ⟶ Ra   Sa ⟶ Ra   **Fig. 17.** The discrimination reversal
    Sb ⟶ Rb   Sb ⟶ Rb   task

the stimulus response pair. For instance, a unit may fire when Sa elicits Ra but not when Sa elicits Rb nor when Ra is elicited by Sb.

The examples given here were oversimplified in that a sensory unit need not respond to one of the stimuli only. It would usually respond to both Sa and Sb but with different response patterns. However, as long as these response patterns depend on the stimuli alone and do not change with the reversal of the responses we consider the unit as sensory.

E. Vaadia studied 147 units in the primary and secondary (belt) auditory areas. In all these recordings the same units were recorded through at least two reversals of response patterns so that changes of response patterns due to some unrelated processes could be ruled out.

Most of the units (92%) responded to the stimuli and most of them responded to both the sine wave (Sa) and the noise (Sb). In all the units the initial response stayed the same thoughout the reversals of response patterns, so that one can state confidently that the initial response of units in the auditory cortex is purely sensory. However, at least 9% of the units showed changes in the later component of the response.

Figure 18 illustrates such a unit. Each frame gives a PST histogram of the unit for different conditions. Press time is when the monkey pressed the lever, 10 ms later a stimulus was turned on, either a pure sine wave at 750 Hz or a band of noise filtered between 712 Hz and 788 Hz. The monkey was trained not to start and move the lever earlier than 300 ms, so that the PST histogram is not contaminated by any sound that might be generated by the movement. Shift time represents the time at which the monkey completed the movement to the left or to the right. At that time the stimulus was turned off and the reward was given. The time from Press to Shift varies from trial to trial, therefore, each PST is divided into two graphs, one triggered around the Press time and one around the Shift time.

If we compare the responses to tone and to noise we see that they are both composed of an off-response but with different time course and amplitude. The responses to the noise stay the same also after reversal of the response pattern. On the other hand the responses to tone look different. When the tone is about to elicit movement to the right (on the top right panel), the cell shows some supression of its firing rate, however, when the tone is about to elicit movement to the left the cell shows a gradual build-up of its firing rate. This increased activity is seen only when movement to the left is elicited by the tone stimulus. The increased firing rate for the association tone → left is not large but highly significant.

As stated earlier, in 9% of the auditory cortex units activity which was related to the sensory motor association was clearly found with the activity being switched on and off with repeated reversals. In another 9% such activity was seen but it was weaker and became statistically significant only if all the respon-

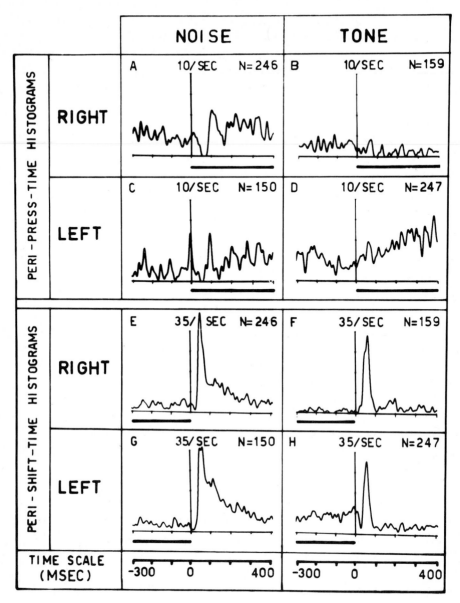

Fig. 18. Responses of a unit during discrimination reversal task.
Each PSTH is made of two parts. *At the top* the rate of firing around the initiation of
the stimulus (*Press*) is plotted. *At the bottom* the rate of firing around the time of completion of movement (*Shift*) is plotted. The sound stimulus was delivered 10 ms after
the Press and continued until the Shift. Reward was administered few hundreds of
milliseconds later. The *tone* stimulus was a 750 Hz pure tone, the *noise* stimulus was a
band pass noise filtered around 750 Hz. The duration of stimulation is marked by the
line under the abscissa. N gives the number of stimuli averaged to construct each histogram. (By courtesy of E. Vaadia)

ses in pattern 1 were pulled together and compared to all the responses in pattern 2. The units with associative activity were distributed equally between the primary and secondary auditory areas (Vaadia et al. 1982).

This study illustrates two points:

a) The same neuron may be involved in different functions at different times.

b) Even in the primary sensory areas nonsensory activity might occur after the initial, sensory-bound activity.

No units with motor components were found. Therefore classification of the auditory area as a sensory area is justified in that most of the units or rather most of the activity of the units is sensory. But these properties do not exclude the possibility that some of the units (9%-18%) exhibit associative activity in addition to their sensory activity.

Furthermore, in the short-term memory experiment of Y. Gottlieb (Chap. 3.2) in which a monkey was trained to compare the pitch of two tones separated by 1 s of silence, 35% of the units showed maintained changes in the firing rate during that 1 s of silence (Fig. 5). During control periods, when the same stimuli were given but the monkey did not respond, this maintained change of firing rate disappeared, indicating that it is associated with the monkey's "will" to memorize the first tone. Although this activity may be classified as sensory activity it is not time-locked in a strict way to the stimulus. In fact, it is present mostly when no physical stimulus is present, during the pause between the two stimuli. Thus, even though most of the units are engaged in sensory processing, the auditory cortex is certainly not just a station through which information is briefly processed and then passed on to other higher stations.

6 Spatio-Temporal Patterns of Activity

6.1 Compound Renewal Densities

When we studied relations between two cells we did not see anything un-expected. We found that two cells may act independently, they may share a common input or they may affect each other synaptically. All these relations could be expected from the known physiology and anatomy. We gained some insight into the cortical connectivity by quantitative analysis of the probability of connections and of the strength of connections, but did not detect any sign of a new type of relation between units. We found that pairs of units work essentially in an independent way and that many diverse sources of excitation (and inhibition) may affect every unit, but we did not see anything that could suggest how the information is coded in the activity of the neural network.

Should we attempt to study also more complex interactions? That de-pends on our model of coding of information within the activity of the neurons. If we think that the relevant parameter is the mode of activity of large populations of neurons, there is little point in studying single units. If we think that for each task there is a specific line in which one strongly excited cell is able to drive another cell strongly, then there is not much use in studying more than the correlation between two cells. If we believe that processing of information involves more complex interactions, then it is worthwhile studying larger groups of cells.

Here we turn the argument around. Since there is no compeling evidence for any of the models, we study the brain with all the techniques described above. If by using one of the techniques we succeed in obtaining evidence that explains adequately some mechanisms of brain function, we tend to believe that the corresponding model is the appropriate one.

In this chapter we shall examine the evidence for the presence of com-plex interactions among neurons. What we wish to do is to study inter-actions within groups of neurons and then if we see only straightforward extension of what is known to exist between pairs of units we would say that cortical processing can be described in terms of a neuron affecting a neuron which affects a neuron, etc. If on the other hand we see some new patterns of activity, we assume that complex patterns of interactions are also involved in processing information. Our studies were limited to interaction among three cells. These studies improved to some extent our ability to analyze interactions between two cells but revealed also, in some cases, complex interactions which up until now could not be seen by studies of interaction in pairs of units.

Let us first discuss the question of how compound interactions among three cells may be studied. Suppose we measured simultaneously the firing times of three neurons A, B, and C (Fig. 19). If we consider only the interaction between neurons B and A we could ask the question what is the expected firing rate of neuron A at time delay t_{BA} after neuron B fired? This expected rate of firing is a function of the interval t_{BA} and was called the cross-renewal density. In a similar manner we could ask how the firing rate of cell A depends on the time (t_{CA}) elapsed from a spike of cell C. In addition to these two cross-renewal densities we could ask more complex questions. We could ask whether the rate of firing of cell A at delay t_{BA} after cell B fired is constant, of perhaps, is it modified also by the firing of neuron C? In a similar fashion we may ask whether the cross renewal of neuron A on neuron C depends also on the firing time of neuron B? In short, we want to ask how the firing rate of neuron A depends jointly on the intervals t_{BA} and t_{CA}.

This three-cell renewal density may be plotted as a three-dimensional graph in which the X-axis is the time elapsed from a spike of neuron B (t_{BA}), the Y-axis is the time elapsed from a spike of neuron C (t_{CA}), and the Z-axis (perpendicular to the plan of the drawing) is the rate of firing of cell A (Fig. 19B). For three cells we may have three such graphs, namely the renewal density of firing of neuron A as a function time elapsed from the firing of neuron B and C, the renewal density of firing of neuron B as a function of time elapsed from the firing of A and C, and, the renewal density of firing of neuron C as a function of time elapsed from the firing of neurons A and B. For these graphs there are only three arguments t_{AC}, t_{BA}, t_{CB}, which are not independent because $t_{CA} = t_{CB} + t_{BA}$. Perkel et al. (1975) suggested a triangular coordinate system for describing this situation. Their triangular system may be obtained by bending our Cartesian coordinate system of figure 19B so that there is 120° between X and Y axes (Fig. 19C). The three renewal densities could then be put together as in Fig. 19D. On this triangular base we could erect a perpendicular axis on which the rate of firing (the renewal density) of the appropriate neuron (A, B, or C) is plotted. In the following graphs this rate is coded in shades of gray and is given as percent of the expected rate (the average rate of the neuron).

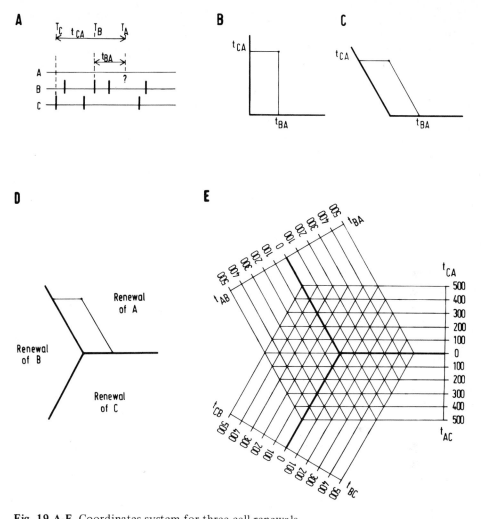

Fig. 19 A-E. Coordinates system for three cell renewals.
A The firing times of neurons B and C are known and the probability of firing of neuron A in relation to these trains is investigated. **B** Regular coordinate system used to plot the firing rate of neuron A as a function of times elapsed from firing of neuron B and neuron C. **C** Same coordinate system as in **B** but the angle between the axes increased to 120°. **D** Three coordinate systems such as in **C** are attached together to give all the possible time relations among the firing of three neurons. **E** The scales of the three axes are projected out and extended to occupy the entire range of the three graphs. The three intervals (t_{CA}, t_{BA}, t_{BC}) associated with any point on the graph can be read by projecting the point onto the three external axes

In order to eliminate the need for plotting the scales inside the graph, the scales are projected outside as seen in Fig. 19E. These projected scales allow one to read all three intervals (t_{CA}, t_{CB}, t_{BA}) associated with each point. For instance, the point shown in Fig. 19D represents the intervals $t_{CA} =$

400 ms, t_{BA} = 200 ms (which imply that t_{CB} is 200 ms), as can be read directly in Fig. 19E.

In reality of course we do not know the renewal densities, but we may estimate them by breaking time into bins and counting the number of spikes in each bin. For the auto- and cross-renewal densities, as well as for the response patterns (PSTH) described earlier, these bins were so small that they were not apparent on the graphs. For the three-cell renewals we do not have enough memory space in the computer to allow for such small bins. Therefore, the graphs are composed of a mosaic of triangular panels. (For technical description of the construction of the renewal densities see Abeles 1982).

6.2 How Three Cells Interact

Let us examine some examples of three cell interactions. In the top half of Fig. 20 we see in a, b, and c the cross-renewal densities between the three pairs of units. Units A and C share a common input, units B and C fire independently, and so do units B and A. The three cells' renewal density is shown below. There is a darker line extending on both sides of the T_A - T_C = 0 axis. This line represents the common input of cells A and C. This dark band looks homogeneous throughout its length, meaning that the strength of common input seen does not depend on the time of firing of the third cell (B), so that the circuit diagram of Fig. 20e may be drawn.

The bottom half of Fig. 20 illustrates a more complex case. The three cross renewals (Fig. 20 f, g, h) show that each pair of cells is driven by a common input. Is there, actually, only one source of input that drives all the three cells, as shown in Fig. 20j, or are there three independent sources each driving one pair only, as shown in Fig. 20k. The three cells' renewal density helps us to choose between the two circuits.

If a common source was driving all three units (Fig. 20j) we expect that each pair will show a stronger synchronization when the third cell fires too. The degree of synchronization between cells A and C, for instance, depends on the strength of their connection with the common input and on the probability of firing of the common input. If instead of averaging their cross-renewal density over all the time we concentrate only on times around which cell B also fired, we increase the chances of obtaining time sections in which the common input fired, and therefore, we expect to see stronger synchronization between cells A and C. Hence, when one common input is driving all three cells we expect to find higher firing rates near the center of the hexagon. Since every band in the three cells renewal is homogeneous throughout its extent (Fig. 20i) we must conclude that we face three independent sources of common input (Fig. 20k).

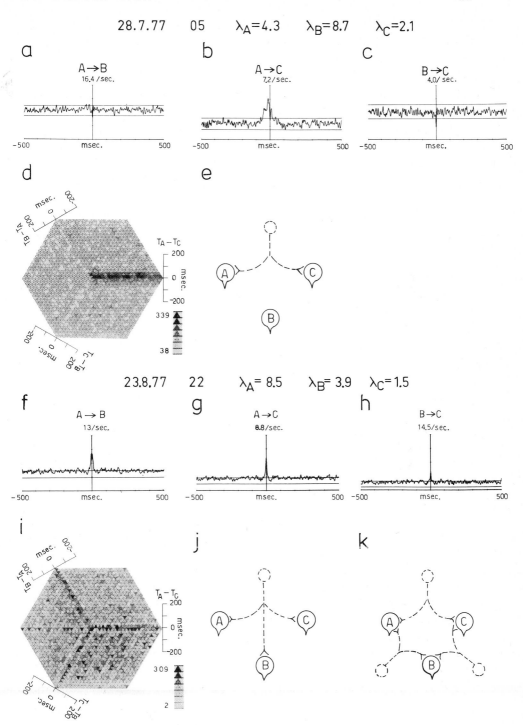

Fig. 20 a-k. Relations among three neurons.
a-e One pair shares a common input. **f-k** Each of the three pairs has a common input

In the cases illustrated so far we did not encounter any unusual interactions. In fact everything has been seen already when we studied the pairs
of cells. This lack of complex interactions is the most common finding in
the three cells renewal analysis, as could be expected from the finding that
most cells have their own way for responding to their input and that interactions, when they exist, are usually quite weak. Figure 21 illustrates an
exception to this rule. Here again cells A and C share a common input resulting in a darker band around $T_A - T_C = 0$ as in Fig. 21d, but this band is
not homogeneous, it is lighter near the center and only at around 200 ms
does it reach the level of the rest of the band. This means that the common
input of neurons A and C is less effective for 200 ms after the firing of
neuron B, indicating that neuron B inhibits the source of common input to
neurons A and C, so that in this case the circuit diagram of Fig. 21e may be
inferred.

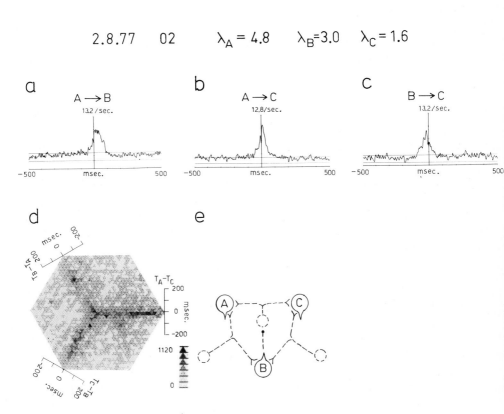

Fig. 21 a-e. Relations among three neurons.
The common input for cell A and C does not produce a homogeneous gray strip around
$T_C - T_A = 0$ line

Although this case illustrates a more complex way for interaction among three cells, it does not indicate any unusual process in the cortex. In 8% (10 out of 129) of the three cell groups we found relations such as in Fig. 22. There, except for the presence of a common input for each pair of cells as seen in the cross-renewal densities of the neurons, we see two dark bins. One near the center and another near $T_4 - T_1 = 375$. This last dark bin means that neuron 5 fires at a high rate within 25 ms after neuron 4 fired, but only when neuron 1 fired 375 ms earlier. In this recording site we could observe the activity of six single units. The triple renewal density of Fig. 22D is based on cells 1, 4, and 5. To visualize the firing patterns associated with the dark bins we plotted the actual firing times of all six units every time a count was added to one of the dark bins. Figure 22E shows these firing patterns. On the left we see the firing of the six cells around the time sequence that corresponds to the center bin of Fig. 22D and on the right we see the firing patterns that corresponds to the bin near the lower left corner of Fig. 22E. Additional examples for such complex firing sequences are shown in Fig. 22F, G, and H.

In all the cases where such special time relations were seen the time delays were quite long — tens to hundreds of milliseconds. How could such a long time delay be accounted for?

One could disregard these complex firing patterns, discarding them as chance events, despite the very low probability of obtaining such relations by chance. (In some cases the probability of obtaining the complex rates by chance was less than 10^{-8} and in no case less than 10^{-6}.) But if we do not wish to discard these observations we face a difficult problem. Time delays of tens or even hundreds of milliseconds must involve a large number of synapses. If one neuron can affect another through dozens of interneurons we must have a chain of interneurons which transmits with almost no failure. It is unlikely that such a long chain in which the activity of one neuron is strictly coupled to that of another exists in the cortex. If such connections did exist we would expect to find at least some cases in our sample where activity of one cell always followed the activity in the other. We never detected in our cross-renewal densities such strong connections at either short or long delays. Even in the case of Fig. 22, in the cross renewal between neurons 1 and 5, there is no indication that neuron 5 tends to fire at a high rate 375 ms after neuron 1 fired. This tendency is seen only when the compound event "neuron 1 fired and 375 ms later neuron 4 fired" is taken into account. Thus we must think of some other arrangement that could result in good-time-locking after many synapses.

A possible arrangement is shown in Fig. 23C. There a set of cells converges on another set of cells which may converge on another set of cells and so on. When the neurons in the first set fire in synchrony, each of the neu-

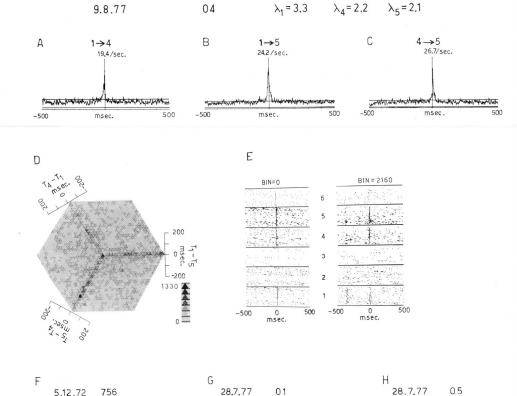

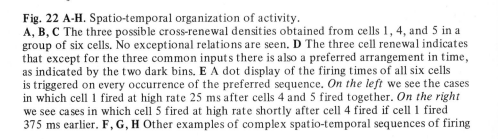

Fig. 22 A-H. Spatio-temporal organization of activity.
A, B, C The three possible cross-renewal densities obtained from cells 1, 4, and 5 in a
group of six cells. No exceptional relations are seen. **D** The three cell renewal indicates
that except for the three common inputs there is also a preferred arrangement in time,
as indicated by the two dark bins. **E** A dot display of the firing times of all six cells
is triggered on every occurrence of the preferred sequence. *On the left* we see the cases
in which cell 1 fired at high rate 25 ms after cells 4 and 5 fired together. *On the right*
we see cases in which cell 5 fired at high rate shortly after cell 4 fired if cell 1 fired
375 ms earlier. **F, G, H** Other examples of complex spatio-temporal sequences of firing

rons in the second set receives synchronous synaptic bombardments which synchronously excite the next set, etc.

This type of arrangement where one set of synchronously firing units excite another set synchronously could maintain time-locking relations over a large number of synapses. The neurons in such a set are ordinary cortical neurons so that they make contacts with and receive contacts from thousands of other cortical cells. Therefore, for each set so activated, there is a large subliminal fringe of neurons all of which receive also excitation at the same time, but this excitation is not strong enough to secure synchronous firing with the rest of the group. When we record from a group of cells and see in their spike trains some specific, complex, time relations we may either be recording from neurons at different stages of such a chain, or from neurons that are indirectly affected (excited or inhibited) by neurons from such a chain. If we happen to record from neurons in the chain, we expect to find very accurate time relations, while if we record from the fringe neurons the time relations are expected to be looser.

If such arrangements exist, why is it that we do not see some locking of activity when we study pairs of neurons? One would expect occasionally to record from a cell which belongs to one set of synchronously firing neurons (or to its subliminal fringe) and from another cell which belongs to a set a few stages down the line. In such a case we would expect to see a clear increase in the firing rate of the other cell at the appropriate delay after the first cell fired. Such relations were never seen. While we found weak, short latency effects which could be attributed to monosynaptic (or perhaps bisynaptic) relations, we did not find long latency time-locking when pairs of neurons were studied.

Why can we see such time-locking after delays of hundreds of milliseconds when we study these cells in triplets? We must conclude that the activity along such a chain of synchronously firing groups occurs only occasionally and that usually excitation is derived from other processes. That is, the chain is not a rigid structure through which activity traverses always in a fixed pattern, but a dynamic entitiy that may be turned on or off according to the spatio-temporal pattern of activity in the cortical network. This concept of dynamic formation and dissolution of functional chains is similar to the "cell assemblies" postulated by Hebb thirty years ago, except for the requirement that the transmission along the chain is secured by the synchronous firing of sets of cells. In these circumstances when we study a pair of neurons from the chain we may observe time-locked activity only occasionally when the chain is functioning. The two neurons are engaged most of the time in other activities which dilute the specific time-locking associated with activity along the chain, making it impossible to discover by two cells correlation techniques. When there are a few neurons associated with the process there is a chance of resolving the activity of the neurons into the occasions related to this chain of synchronous firing and into other processes.

Let us use a numerical example to illustrate this point. Assume that occasionally when the activity is organized along a certain chain cell 1 fires, then after 50 ms cell 2 fires and after additional 25 ms cell 3 fires. If we measure the cross-renewal density between cells 2 and 3 we may not observe a significant peak at 25 ms delay because the activity in the chain is infrequent. But if instead of using all the spikes of cell 2 to estimate this cross-renewal density, we use only those spikes of cell 2 which came 50 ms after the firing of cell 1, we sort out most of the spikes of cell 2 which are not related to the activity along the chain. Hence, we have a good chance to detect a peak in the firing rate of cell 3 25 ms later.

The suggestion that activity is organized along chains of synchronously firing groups of neurons is new and we must ask two questions to evaluate it:(a) To what extent do the known anatomy and physiology support the possibility of such an organization? (b) Is there any reason to believe that this type or organization of activity has any special significance for the processing of information in the cortex? I shall attempt to show in the next chapter that the answer to both questions is in the affirmative.

7 Transmission of Information by Coincidence

In the previous chapters we reached the following conclusions: Each nerve cell receives from and gives contacts to many neurons. Even cells which are close together usually recieve different sources of excitation and inhibition, both when the spontaneous and when the sensory evoked activities are considered. The sensory input is organized so that the units in any certain region of the cortex tend to be affected more by some sort of stimuli and less by others, however, the details of the responses are such that we must assume that many independent sensory inputs converge into the same region.

The independence of the various driving sources reaching a group of neurons results in very little coherence of the firing times of the neurons in the group. The activity of a single neuron shows very little structure. Except for a short refractoriness (seen in all neurons) and a slight tendency for increased excitability immediately after the refractory period (seen in most cells) the firing looks like a random Poisson process.

Only while studying interaction among three neurons did we occasionally see specific structure in the firing sequence which could be described in the following manner: when neuron A fires and after some specific delay T_1 neuron B fires, only then, after some additional delay T_2 does neuron C have a high probability of firing. The delays, T_1 and T_2, could reach several hundreds of milliseconds (450 ms was the largest observed). This type of time-locking could be explained by assuming that neural activity is largely organized in the form of synchronously firing sets of neurons. Each set excites synchronous firing in the next set, which in turn excite synchronously the next set of neurons, etc. We shall call this arrangement of synchronously firing sets, which will be discussed more fully in Sections 7.2 and 7.3, the *synfire chain*. Each synfire chain is activated only occasionally, so that most of the time the firing of any individual neuron may not be associated with one particular chain.

In the previous chapters we computed the connectivity and the strength of contacts in the cortical network. Is the existence of such chains of synchronously firing neurons compatible with these connectivity figures?

7.1 The Single Neuron as a Coincidence Detector

The classical way of looking at a neuron is to view it as an integrator.
This view, as suggested by Sherrington (1906) and proven by direct measurements from motoneurons of the spinal cord (Eccles 1957), says that all the currents generated by the synaptic bombardments of dendrites and soma add up to determine the membrane potential of the cell body. The body is essentially equipotential and its potential is also very close to that of the axon hillock and initial segment of the axon which are the most sensitive areas. When the potential there reaches threshold the neuron fires a spike that goes down its axon and axonal branches to affect other neurons.

Our analysis of the membrane potential fluctuations, the threshold and the excitability of the cortical neuron (Chap. 3) was based on that view. We assumed, there, that each neuron integrates the excitatory and inhibitory effects of 20,000 neurons and that the resulting fluctuations of intracellular membrane potential cause it to fire at 5 spikes per second in a random fashion. On this background of ongoing processes any additional excitatory input will depolarize the cell a little and increase its excitability. We suggested two ways to measure the strength of synaptic contact between two cells. First we asked how many spikes would be evoked in the postsynaptic neuron by a single presynaptic spike? This was computed and found to be 0.003 postsynaptic spikes per presynaptic spike. This is the figure to be used when we wish to study the effects of several asynchronously firing cells. If we wished to increase the firing rate of the cell from 5 spikes to 6 spikes per second we would have to add 333 excitatory inputs arriving asynchronously during that second. Note that this synaptic strength is a marginal strength based on the already existing background firing. Had there been no ongoing excitatory activity we would need many more asynchronously firing excitatory inputs to get an extra spike.

The other way to look at the strength of a presynaptic source was to ask: what is the ratio between the threshold (T) and the amplitude (A) of the EPSP generated by that source? This T/A ratio was found, under the same assumptions, to be 29. In other words, 29 simultaneous presynaptic excitatory spikes are needed to bring the average membrane potential to threshold. It seems that coincident firing is about 10 times more efficient than asynchronous integrated activity. Higher efficiency of coincident activity was found also experimentally in studies of cross-renewal density where on the average a presynaptic spike could evoke 0.06 spikes but the ratio of threshold to the EPSP amplitude was 7 (see Chap. 4.3 for discussion of the discrepancy between the experimental and anatomical estimates).

We conclude that although the neuron operates as an integrator it is especially sensitive to coincident firing of a few presynaptic sources. Coming back to the synfire chain suggested in the previous section, it is evident that activity within a network of neurons would tend to organize itself in chains of synchronously firing groups if the proper connections exist.

7.2 Existence of Chains of Neuronal Sets With Appropriate Connections

Is it likely that the cortical network contains sets of neurons wired in the appropriate way to support activity in chains of synchronously firing sets? The simplest view of such an arrangement is given in Fig. 23C. The sets there are made of three neurons each, connected in such a way that each cell in one set excites every cell in the next set down the line, so that each cell on the second set receives excitatory inputs from all three neurons of the previous set. Such an arrangement could go on and on to generate a chain of sets in which each of the neurons in one set excites all the neurons in the next one.

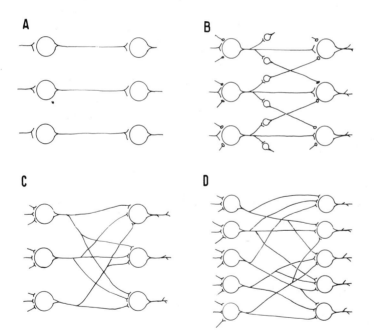

Fig. 23 A-D. Schematic representation of neural chains.
A One-to-one chain. **B** One-to-one chain with lateral inhibition. **C** Synfire chain. Each neuron in one stage excites every neuron in the next stage. **D** Modified synfire chain. Each of the five neurons in one stage excites three neurons of the next stage

A set of three neurons seems very small in the sense that very strong synapses are required to secure the transmission of synchronously firing from one set to another. However, if such connectivity exists also for larger sets of 20 to 40 neurons per set, then this type of activity will always be present in the cortex because in each cubic millimeter of cortex during every millisecond, on the average, 200 neurons fire (40,000 neurons/mm³ x 5 spikes/neuron/s x 0.001 s).

We take again the anatomical connectivity assumed earlier, that is that each neuron contacts 8000 other neurons within a cube of 1 x 1 x 1 mm, and ask the following question:

Assume we pick up N neurons (that fired synchronously) what is the probability that there will exist around them another set of at least N neurons contacted by the first set as in Fig. 23C? That is, each neuron in the second set receives a synapse from each of the neurons in the first set. This probability depends, of course, on the size (N) of the set. If for instance, we know that two neighboring neurons fired together then there are on the average 1600 neurons around them, each of which receives synapses from both neurons, because the first neuron affects 40,000 x 0.2 neurons, and 0.2 of these are affected also by the other neuron. Hence the probability of finding at least two neurons which receive synaptic contacts from both (firing) neurons is practically one. If, on the other hand, we know that ten neighboring neurons fired together, then we expect to find only 40,000 x 0.2^{10} (= 0.004) neurons which receive contacts from all the ten (firing) neurons. In these circumstances the probability of finding at least ten neurons, each of which receive contacts from all the ten (firing) neurons, is practically zero. In a generalized form we ask the following question: If we chose a set of N neurons, what is the probability of finding at least N other neurons each of which is connected to each of the neurons from the first set? Figure 24 shows this probability as a function of N. For very small sets the probability is very close to one, for large sets it is very close to zero and the changeover from one to zero is very sharp, at five neurons per set.

The cortical network contains the proper connections for such chains of sets of neurons. However, the neural activity will not become organized along these chains unless the synapses are strong enough to assure the transmission of synchronous firing down the chain without dissipation. The average synapse is far too weak for that. One needs to strengthen the synapses from their average strength of 29 (threshold to EPSP ratio) to less than 5 in order to establish a functioning synfire chain. Examination of Fig. 24 shows that around the strength of 5 there is a sharp transition from nonfunctioning to functioning synfire chains, so that if the neurophysiological basis of learning is the strengthening of synapses and learned tasks are carried via synfire chains, then there would be a critical strength below which a learned task cannot be executed. This is one of the properties that make the synfire chain an attractive candidate for information transmission and processing at the higher levels of the nervous system. But, before considering the functional significance of the arrangement of activity in such synfire chains we should make some technical comments on the estimate of the size of the sets made here.

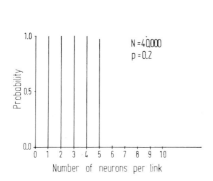

Fig. 24. Probability of existence of a synfire link.

We compute here the probability of the following trial: Pick N neurons within a small cortical volume, what is the probability of finding around them other N neurons, each of which is connected to every one of the N neurons we picked? (Fig. 23C illustrates such a link for N = 3). Probabilities were computed by first finding the expected number of neurons on which N neurons make contacts ($X = 40'000 \cdot (0.2)^N$), and then computing the probability of obtaining at least N such post-synaptic neurons (given the expected number X)

The figure of five neurons per set should not be taken too strictly. It depends on the connectivity within the cortex and depends also on the form of connections between the sets. Figure 23D represents another possible arrangement, there the sets are five cells wide, each neuron in the second set receives synaptic contacts from three cells out of the five in the first set. If one allows for such arrangements one obtains different figures for the sets' size. However, two basic properties stay invariable: such cortical networks exist even in a random network so that there is no need to assume specific growth patterns during embryogenesis, and the average synaptic strength is too weak and must be increased in order to support transmission of synchronous volleys down the synfire chain.

7.3 Some Properties of Synfire Chains

Let us compare the properties of such chains of synchronously firing cells with those of a simple chain of neurons. At the peripheral sensory system we often think of a stimulus that comes in, and excites the receptor cells, which in turn excite the first-order neuron, which sends its axon into the brain to make a strong synaptic contact with a relay neuron, and so on.

This type of arrangement is presented schematically in Fig. 23A. There activity is relayed from one cell to another through very strong synapses. At each stage there are many neurons whose properties may vary along some continous variable: pitch of sound, place in visual field or place on the body. This kind of arrangement will be termed transmission by *dedicated line*. The dedicated line arrangement in sensory systems is often coupled with a lateral inhibitory arrangement (Fig. 23B), which serves to sharpen boundaries and reduce the size of the receptive field (Hartline et al. 1956).

The synfire chain is arranged as in Fig. 23C or D, so that transmission from stage to stage is secured by the synchronous firing of all the cells in one stage.

Let us compare some of the properties of the two modes of transmission.

a) *Code.* In the dedicated line arrangement the simplest code is the firing rate of the cell. If one cell fires a burst of spikes at a high rate, it will excite strongly the next cell along the line which will then fire a burst of spikes and so on.

In the synfire chain the code is synchrony of firing among the members of the same set. Under normal circumstances one would expect that each cell in a set when activated synchronously by the cells from the previous set will also generate a burst of spikes. But the burst is not the important parameter of the code.

b) *Receptive Fields.* In the dedicated line the size of the peripheral receptive field is preserved along the line or could be reduced if lateral inhibitions are present.

In the synfire chain, the diverging and converging pattern of connectivity blurs out the receptive field of the individual neuron.

c) *Topographic Arrangement.* The mapping of the receptor surface in the periphery (retina, cochlea, body surface) tends to be preserved by the dedicated lines. The synfire chain tends to mix up this arrangement (see also property g).

d) *Multifunction.* A neuron in a dedicated line can be used to transmit information in one type of processing only. Two dedicated lines cannot cross over (as in Fig. 25A) because once the cross-over point is excited there is no way to tell which way the activity will proceed. In the synfire chain the same neuron may participate in many different chains according to whether it fires synchronously with one set of cells or with another. Figure 25B illustrates this situation. What appears at first glance as a tangle of connections is representing, partially, two synfire chains. When synchronous excitation enters the network, from the top left end it will propagate in three stages and appear from the bottom right end as a synchronous volley. Similarly, synchronous activity, coming from the bottom left end, will come out from upper right end synchronously. The neurons of each synfire chain are marked by stripes in a different direction to facilitate their identification. The cross-hatched neurons participate in both chains. By following the interconnections it will become evident that when either synfire chain is active most neurons in the network are affected. It is only by directing our attention to the internal synchronization of firing among the neurons that we can distinguish which of the two synfire chains is active.

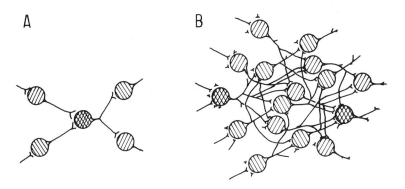

Fig. 25 A, B. Cross-over of neural chains.
A Cross-over of two one-to-one chains. Functionally such a cross-over is not possible. Therefore, each brain process must have its own dedicated chain. **B** Cross-over of two synfire chains. Such a cross-over can function as long as the two chains are not active simultaneously

e) *Immunity to Damage.* The dedicated line is very sensitive to failure of individual neurons. If one neuron in a chain dies, all the chain becomes useless. This vulnerability becomes serious when long chains of neurons are considered. If, for example, some simple neural process lasting 0.5 s is carried by a chain of 500 neurons exciting each other as in Fig. 23 A, then after 1 year with a neuronal fallout of 0.5% per year its probability of staying intact is less than 0.0092! The synfire chain, especially if arranged as in Fig. 23D, is not affected by loss of some neurons here and there. It will be affected only when several neurons of the same link fall out — a very unlikely event for links made up of small number of neurons.

f) *Parallel Processing.* The dedicated lines do not cross over (d. above), therefore for each type of processing there must exist a separate line. This allows for activation of many processes simultaneously with little interference between processes.

The synfire chains could be activated in parallel only if they utilize separate sets of neurons. If they share the same neurons (as in Fig. 25B) there is a danger that activity set up by one chain would render these common neurons refractory when needed by the other chain.

g) *Localization.* Transmission of sensory information in the periphery is carried out by stages, each of which is localized in different anatomical structures. This type of segregation may be continued all throughout the cortex by dedicated lines. On the other hand sets of neurons in a synfire chain are likely to be distributed in a quasirandom mode. Thus, the structure of stages of Fig. 23C and D. Fig. 25B and Fig. 31 represent the time of activation along the chain and *not the anatomical position.*

Anatomically, if we look at a region in which such synfire transmission occurs, we are likely to see pictures such as in Fig. 26. There, one hundred cells are represented by dots in a 10 x 10 matrix. The cells seem to fire at random times, but if relations between units are studied we may see that all the cells marked by a fire together, after that cells marked by b fire, then c and so on. All the cells marked a belong to one link in a synfire chain, all the cells marked b belong to the next link and so on. The propagation of synchronous activity down the chain is not associated here with clear topographic shift of excitation. Anatomically, the activity may appear distributed evenly across the network or may be associated with statistical drift of the center of gravity of active cells. In Fig. 26 such a drift from the upper-left to the lower-right region is seen. There is no reason why the same neuron would not participate in the chain at two (b and x) or more stages.

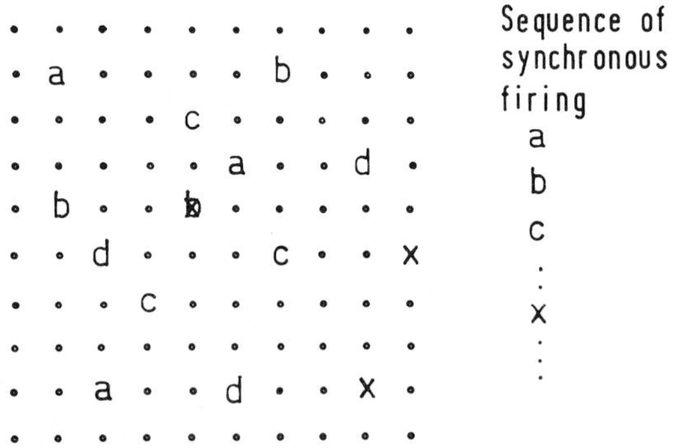

Fig. 26. Appearance of synfire activity within a population of neurons.
The order of the synfire chains of Fig. 23 and 25 is given to stress the functional relations. Anatomically the links of the synfire chain may be distributed quasi-randomly. If one could see the activity in the cortex while a synfire chain is active, one might see spatio-temporal organization of activity as drawn here

Although the two alternatives, *dedicated lines* and *synfire chains* were exposed here as two distinct categories there exist a whole spectrum of intermediate structures. By adding more and more collaterals to a dedicated line structure such as in Fig. 23A one moves gradually towards a synfire chain such as in Fig. 23D.

We arrived at the idea of synfire chains by the observation of complex spatio temporal patterns of activity in groups of three neurons. Could one observe the synfire chain from another angle? The answer is yes: when a large proportion of the spontaneously firing of neurons is organized in synfire chains this organization affects the surface recorded electrocorticogram (ECoG). These effects will be described in the next chapter.

8 Organization of Generators of the ECoG

8.1 The Generation of the ECoG

There exists a vast literature dealing with the mechanisms of electrocorticogram (ECoG) generation (e.g., Elul 1972, Creutzfeldt 1974). This section summarizes the main points required for understanding the statistics of population to be developed in the next section.

The ECoG waveform is statistically similar to the intracellular membrane fluctuations that are recorded from cortical neurons. By statistical similarity we mean that the amplitude fluctuations have a similar power spectrum both in the ECoG and in the intracellular records and that as this power spectrum changes, while the animal falls asleep or wakes up, both the ECoG and the intracellular membrane fluctuations change in the same way. Therefore, the ECoG is thought to be generated by summation of synaptic activities over many cortical cells. The pyramidal cells are the most effective contributors because their structure permits the generation of potential difference between the apical dendrites and the basal dendrites. Such potential differences are equivalent to a large dipole (0.5-1.5 mm long) standing perpendicular to the cortical surface. An electrode placed on the surface may be affected by the activity of some 100,000 pyramidal neurons. If the activity of all these units is completely chaotic there will be no appreciable surface recording. This was shown by Elul (1972) who carefully injected small doses of tetrodotoxin, thereby manging to block all firing from deep brain structures without affecting the cortical cells. Under such conditions many of the cortical cells continued to fire but no voltage waves were recorded from the surface. Hence, some degree of synchronization between the activity of cortical units must exist in order to generate an appreciable ECoG.

We may think of each pyramidal neuron as a generator contributing its small share to the electric potential at the surface. This contribution is governed by the physics of electric fields in a volume conductor (Plonsey 1977), by the morphology of the pyramidal neurons, and by the distribution of potentials along their dendritic tree. These factors are too complex to be analyzed quantitatively, but for our purpose it is sufficient to assume that at each point we obtain an algebraic sum of the contribution of all the generators around that point.

The way the generators add up depends on the statistic relations among them. If all the generators were synchronized the Root-Mean-Square (RMS) amplitude of the summed activity would be much bigger than the amplitude of an individual generator. If there were 100,000 such generators, the amplitude of the completely synchronized population would be 100,000 times bigger, while if the activity of the generators was uncorrelated the summed activity would be only $\sqrt{100,000} = 316$ times bigger than the amplitude of the individual generator.

As stated earlier, there must exist some degree of synchronization among the generators or else their effects cancel out to extent that only a very small wave will be recorded. The form and source of this synchronization is still a matter of controversy. As we saw in the previous chapters, in the awake cortex there is only little synchronization between the firing times of pairs of neurons. When we recorded from several pairs, though each pair could show signs of common drive, they were driven by different and independent sources. This can be interpreted as evidence that in the cortex one can find many local processes, each of which activates some fraction of the neurons. We look for experimental ways to estimate the number of such processes in a given brain area.

8.2 Population Statistics and ECoG

As discussed in the previous section, at any given point the potential is the summed activity of all the generators around it. However, when a macro-electrode is placed over the tissue, it *averages* the potential from all the points under it. Thus, if we increase the size of the recording electrode we average the potential from more and more points, and thereby average the potential of more and more generators.

If all the generators were active in an asynchronous way we would expect to see this averaged potential falling off as the square root of the number of generators. While if all the generators are synchronized we should get a constant amplitude at all electrode sizes. This prediction suggests the following experiment.

Measure the ECoG simultaneously from several electrodes of different sizes. From each electrode compute the mean squared amplitude (variance) of the recorded voltage and plot it against one over the electrode's area. In Fig. 27 we see the expected results of this experiment for the two extreme types of relationships among generators. If all the generators were synchronized we should obtain a constant amplitude at all the electrode sizes. It is hard to evaluate this amplitude, but it should be of the same order of magnitude as the ECoG during an epileptic seizure, that is a few millivolts. If all the generators were desynchronized we should get a straight line going down to zero for infinitely big electrodes.

In reality far-away structures are expected to contribute some common waveform to all the recording points. This common pattern will stay constant at all electrode sizes. In this way the common pattern contributes the same amount of variance to all the electrodes and raises the entire curve.

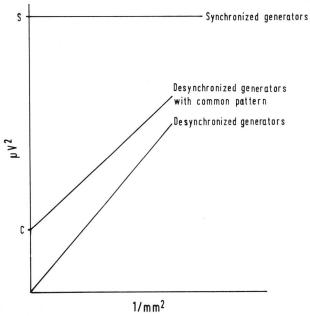

Fig. 27. Amplitude of ECoG recorded through electrodes of different sizes – a theoretical analysis

A similar effect will be seen if a common pattern of waveform is spread over large areas of the brain. Such patterns could be generated by thalamic nuclei that spread their effect over large cortical areas. Their effect may be manifested in having under each unit area a certain fraction of neurons which are driven only by the activity coming from these deep nuclei, or having each neuron affected partially by this activity, or any intermediate arrangement.

All these possibilities have the common property that at each point the recorded EEG may be broken into two waveforms. The first one is a common pattern spread over large areas of the cortex, while the other part represents the summed activity of many uncorrelated local processes. In all these situations, when the total variance (mean squared amplitude) of the ECoG is plotted against the reciprocal of the electrode size, we should obtain a straight line which crosses the ordinate at the level of the variance of the common pattern.

The slope of the line represents the number of new independent generators which are added per unit increase in electrode size. It depends also on the amount contributed by each independent source to the ECoG. If the common pattern is due to activity of some remote brain structures these two factors (density of independent sources of activity and the amplitude of individual source) remain the same and we should have a line parallel to what we would obtain for completely desynchronized generators. If, on the other hand, the common pattern is due to processes internal to the population of generators the graph becomes flatter. If a bigger fraction of the generators is synchronized the graph will become even flatter, reaching the horizontal line when all the generators are synchronized.

This simple case, where all the generators of the ECoG are synchronized, is the extreme case of the common pattern in which no independent new sources are added with increasing size of electrode and, therefore, the slope of the line graph is zero.

A different type of graph is expected if the activity is organized in groups of neurons synchronized among each other. In this case, the total population of the neurons may be divided into many smaller subpopulations within which the activity is synchronized, but the activity of any one subpopulation is uncorrelated with that of any other subpopulation. Let us assume, for the time being, that the members of these subpopulations are not concentrated topographically, but are scattered in a random fashion throughout the cortex. As we record from larger and larger electrodes our ECoG becomes the averaged activity of more and more generators. When a small electrode is increased in size, any additional generators recruited to the recording are likely to belong to different subpopulations and therefore their activity is likely to cancel out some of the activity of neurons from other subpopulations. Therefore, at small electrode sizes the existence of such subpopulations is not evident and the graph looks as predicted for completely desynchronized generators. However, if the electrodes are very large any further increase will not recruit any new independent generators, instead we recruit more generators which are synchronized with the ones we have already seen with the smaller electrodes. At this stage increasing the electrode size does not reduce the amplitude of the ECoG any more.

We expect to obtain a graph such as in Fig. 28. From this graph the number of subpopulations in the cortex under the electrode may be estimated in the follogwing manner: Let us denote by S the amplitude we would get if all the generators were completely synchronized. If we have N independent subpopulations then at large electrode sizes the amplitude of the ECoG should level off at $P = S/N$, because S represents the variance of the single generator and P represents the variance of the average obtained from N independent processes.

When we add to the ECoG some common widespread component we simply shift the whole line up by an amount equivalent to the mean square amplitude of that common widespread wave. As in the case of completely desynchronized population the slope of the linear part of the graph will not change if the common wave is added to the ECoG and will flatten if it is generated by partial common activity of the neurons in the region.

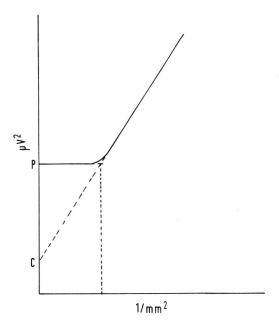

Fig. 28. Amplitudes of ECoG recorded through electrodes of different sizes. Theoretical analysis for ECoG generated by several subpopulations of neurons. In each subpopulation the activity is synchronized but the various populations are uncorrelated

The last possibility to be considered is the existence of topographical organization. The brain cortex is made up of areas with different connections and variable functions. If the electrode size becomes very large it may cover a mixture of regions. At smaller electrode sizes while we are above one region we may record a graph that flattens off such as in Fig. 28, but as the electrodes become very big they recruit generators from other regions

containing new subpopulations and the graph starts to fall off again as in
Fig. 29. From the initial part of the curve we can still compute the number
of subpopulations and from the turning point of the curve we can obtain the
size of the area within which they are distributed.

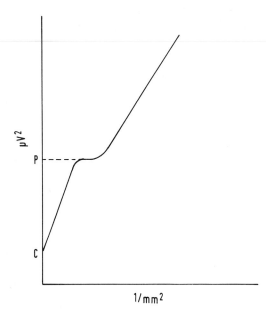

Fig. 29. Amplitude of ECoG through
electrodes of different sizes.
Theoretical analysis for ECoG generated as in Fig. 28 but only in a limited brain area

In summary, studies of the relation between ECoG amplitude and electrode size may teach us something about the way by which the activities of
the neurons in the cortex are related to each other.

8.3 Experimental Results

In order to make recordings of the type discussed in the previous section
A. Arieli performed a series of experiments in which he recorded the ECoG
through an array of concentric electrodes (Fig. 30A). The electrodes were
made of a 10 μ-thick gold layer printed over a silicone rubber sheet. When
placed over the exposed cortex they adhere to the surface by capillary
forces and assure a good but flexible contact.

When the ECoG of unanesthetized, but paralyzed cats was recorded
through this electrode array (against an indifferent electrode on the cat's
neck), ECoG's such as in Fig. 30B were seen. As predicted by the theoretical considerations the smallest (No. 7) electrode recorded the ECoG with

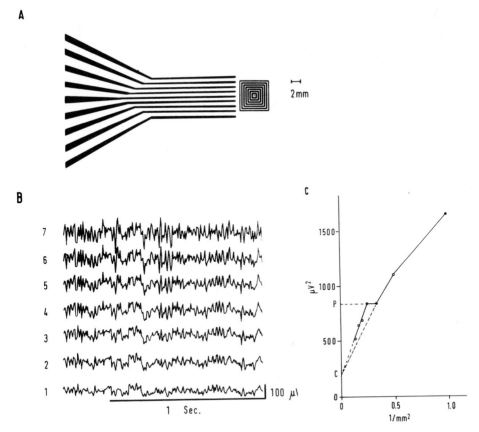

Fig. 30 A-C. Amplitude of ECoG as recorded through concentric electrodes. **A** The electrode array-printed on silastic sheet. Only the squares were in contact with the brain. **B** Sample of the recorded ECoG. 7 is recorded from the inner square and *1* from the outer square. **C** ECoG amplitude against electrode size. (By courtesy of A. Arieli)

highest amplitudes. When the mean squared amplitude of such a recording was plotted against the reciprocal of electrode size the graph of Fig. 30 C was obtained. The bend in the graph is real, it was obtained with two sets of electrodes placed at eight different orientations over the same region.

By extrapolating the three segments of the curve back to zero (infinitely large electrodes) we obtain the following estimates: The region containing statistical homogeneous properties extends to electrodes 3 or 4, covering a square area of 3 x 3 to 4 x 4 mm. The graph flattens off at 800 μV^2. As the electrode covers more than 4 x 4 mm it recruits more and more independent sources and the amplitude declines again toward a common waveform of 200 μV^2.

The number of independent groups of neurons in the 3.5 x 3.5 mm square may be evaluated in the following way. The amplitude of ECoG expected if all the generators were synchronized is about 3 mV. Thus, the mean squared amplitude of a completely synchronized population (S) is 9,000,000 μV^2. The level of saturation (P-C) is 600 μV^2, therefore, the number of subpopulations is N = 9,000,000/600 = 15,000. These populations are distributed over a cortical area of about 3.5 x 3.5 = 12.25 mm^2. An area this size will contain about 500,000 pyramidal cells (we count only pyramidal cells because we think that they contribute to the surface ECoG much more than stellate cells). Thus, on the average each subpopulation contains 500,000 : 15,000 = 33 pyramidal cells.

The estimates are very sensitive to the voltage and diameter estimates as they go by the square of these figures. Therefore, the experiments have to be repeated with different electrode configurations, at different brain areas and under different physiological conditions.

The main points illustrated by these experiments are that statistical organization of the neural activity can be studied without the need to monitor explicitly the activity of many thousands of neurons simultaneously, and that there is evidence for the parcellation of the overall cortical activity into small groups of synchronously firing neurons.

9 Information Codes for Higher Brain Function

It seems that we have collected enough data to try and state explicitly our hypothesis about coding and processing of information at the higher levels of the brain. We assume that this code is carried out somehow by the electric activity of neurons and shall discuss the question of how this activity codes the information.

Currently, there are two prevailing views — the dedicated line and the mass action hypotheses. To these we add here the synfire chain hypothesis. This chapter defines briefly these three hypotheses, it describes how the main known properties fit these hypotheses and how they dictate the type of experiments to conduct.

9.1 Hypotheses

a) *Dedicated Line:* For each process there is a line of neurons that excite one another very strongly. The code is, therefore, which cells fire at high rates. Many neurophysiologists, however, would prefer to state that for each neuron in the cortex there exists some appropriate process that will make if fire at a high rate (the adequate stimulus), rather than commit themselves to the dedicated line terminology.

It is usually assumed that as we move away from the periphery (sensory or motor) there will be only a few cells involved in each process. In perceptual processes each entity might have its own representative cells — for instance *grandmother* neurons that fire vigorously only when one sees his own grandmother. Despite this specificity, due to the large connectivity of the cortical neuron, each such specific neuron will excite weakly many other neurons. Therefore, each neuron may be excited weakly by several stimuli but it has also its own specific adequate stimulus that would make it fire vigorously.

At the motor end of the process there are "command neurons" for certain types of movements. These commands are then spelled out by the motor systems (motor cortex, basal ganglia, cerebellum, and spinal cord) into a series of coordinated contractions of muscles. Thus, at the motor end the dedicated line is actually a divergent set of lines in which the appropriate command cell activates, through several stages, many motor neurons of the appropriate muscles.

In a similar fashion at the sensory end we have a succession of converging connections. Simple peripheral receptive fields converge upon neurons which are sensitive to certain simple features of the stimulus. Such simple features are added together to make more complex feature detectors and so on (e.g., Hubel and Wiesel 1962). The two systems must be connected by a complex switchboard. At the switchboard level single, or a few, sensory detectors are connected through a dedicated line to one, or a few, command neurons. In principle, each sensory detector may be connected to every command neuron. The exact connection made depends on the animal experience in the past and on the circumstances preceding the stimulus.

Although the description is given in terms of a stimulus-response paradigm, the idea is carried over to other high-level functions of the cortex. Each element of memory, thought, or feeling has its own groups of neurons which are activated when that element is active and conversely whenever the neurons representing a certain memory (or thought) fire at high rates that means that this memory (or thought) is active.

b) *Mass Action.* According to this hypothesis (John 1967, 1972) the activity of a single neuron is of little importance for coding information. Instead it is the envelope of the summed activity of very large populations of neurons that counts. For each process several populations are activated, each having its own modes of activity. The interference pattern that arises among these modes determines the response of the animal.

Each of these populations is thought to be concentrated topographically in one brain area; one can thereby measure the mode of activity of the population by recording the activity through a gross electrode placed over the area containing the neurons. In a few special cases the ways by which the activity of the population are reflected in the surface recording have been analyzed (e.g., Freeman 1975, Mitzdorf and Singer 1978). Usually, such gross potential changes cannot be translated into patterns of firing of the underlying neurons, but their main property is that different modes of activity of the neurons will add up to generate different forms of recorded wave shapes and thus lend themselves to experimental monitoring.

c) *Synfire Chain.* This has been discussed extensively in the previous chapters. According to this hypothesis the activity of the neurons that transmit information is organized along a chain of sets of neurons. Each link in the chain is made of a set of neurons that fire in exact synchrony whenever the chain becomes active. Neurons of each set converge on neurons of the next and therefore, synchronized activity of one set elicit synchronized activity in the next set and so on. Although the activity of each neuron in the chain is likely to be organized in a short burst, the relevant code is the combination of neurons that fire in synchrony.

The size of each set in a synfire chain is small but there is a large subsynchronous fringe of neurons affected by the activity in the chain. A single neuron may be affected by many synfire chains and may even be a part of several synfire chains (Figs. 25, 26, 31).

9.2 Experimental Evidence

Unfortunately, there has been no decisive experimental evidence to prove or rule out any of these three hypotheses, although the amount of relevant observations is huge. No attempt to review this vast literature is made here, instead just a few experimental facts will be brought forth in connection with each of the hypotheses.

The dedicated line hypothesis draws support from the finding that neurons of the visual cortex respond best to lines or edges at a certain orientation (Hubel and Wiesel 1962). This is taken as proof for the existence of feature detectors as required by the dedicated line hypothesis. The hypothesis is also supported by the existence of a neurons that fires extensively when a monkey intends to reach for an object with its hand — the command neurons, such as was described by Mountcastle et al. (1975). Such neurons do not fire when the monkey moves its hand for purposes other than reaching an object. They also do not respond to the presence of an object if the monkey does not intend to reach it. Their activity does not depend simply on the place in space to which the monkey reaches, but only on the purpose of the movement which is reaching. Such units thus represent a feature of movement generators.

It is rather disturbing that despite the huge experimental effort put into single-unit recordings, the attempts to discover cortical units with complex features (such as *grandmother*) have failed. This may be due to the absence of such feature detectors in the cortex (the best example in noncortical areas is feature detectors for food in the lateral hypothalamus found by (Rolls 1978) or may be because the dedicated line hypothesis is correct only at the periphery of the nervous system. Usually, it is claimed that there are so many complex features that the chances of finding the right feature for the neuron we happen to record from is almost zero.

Although the classical view of the sensory systems is that at the periphery they are organized in dedicated lines, some important exceptions to this rule were found out in the last years. The code for smell (and taste) in the periphery does not reside in specific receptors for few primary odors (or tastes) but in the cross-fiber profile of activity elicited by each stimulus.

In this way even the simplest analysis of stimulus calls for extensive inter-actions between the incoming sensory fibers (Erickson and Schiffman 1975). The perception of complex sounds at moderate and high intensities cannot be based on the selectivity of the auditory fibers to frequencies of sound. At such intensities most of the fibers within the frequency band of the stimulus fire at their maximal possible rate. The code for pitch in these circumstances must be contained in the timing of spikes at the various auditory fibers (Young and Sachs 1979).

The mass action hypothesis is supported by two types of experiments. In the first type a cat is trained to discriminate between a train of flashes at 10 per second and one at 6 per second. When the ECoG is recorded while the cat performs the task, one may find that in many cortical (and subcorti-cal) areas, as the cat makes a mistake, confusing the 6-per-second train with the 10-per-second train, the ECoG wave oscillates at 10 per second instead of 6 per second (John and Killam 1960). Another type of support is drawn from human scalp recordings in which slow waves may be associated with mental processes. Such are the contingent negative variation (CNV), a slow negative wave developing when a subject prepares himself to receive a stimu-lus (Walter 1964), or the positive 300 (P300), a slow positive wave reaching its peak 300 ms after a subject received a stimulus about the nature of which he was in doubt before receiving it (e.g., Donchin et al. 1975).

While these experiments indicate that some special processes take place in the cortex at the time of the slow surface waves, they certainly do not prove that it is the envelope of all the activitiy that counts. The neurons in the cortex have by and large steady response properties. Even when small groups of neurons are considered (Chap. 5) each neuron has its own stable appropriate stimuli and its own stable response pattern. It is not clear why the brain needs to average the responses of millions of neurons which in no way look like a uniform population.

It is also not clear how this type of code operates when we do not face a well-defined point in time to which the process may be locked. Although the ongoing ECoG may be thought of as representing the mode of ongoing activity in the cortex, in the awake state the activity of the units is almost uncorrelated (Chap. 4) so that there is little statistical justification for speaking about the mode of activity.

The synfire chain hypothesis is new and has the least direct experimen-tal support. The main experimental support described here are the findings that the same neuron may participate at different times in different func-tions, sensory and associative, (Chap. 5.4), that during spontaneous activity well-defined complex patterns involving delays of over 100 ms are found (Chap. 6), and the ability to factor the ECoG into some 15,000 processes each associated with only a few neurons (Chap. 9). Strict synchronization between pairs of units has been described for the visual cortex by Toyama (1978).

The main difficulties in accepting the synfire chain hypothesis are the lack of experimental evidence for the use that the brain makes of the synfire chain and the need to translate the code at the periphery into a synfire code. At the periphery, both sensory or motor, the code in most cases is composed of firing rates of neurons organized along some topographic map. If central processing is done by synfire chains, then the place and firing rate code at the sensory end needs to be translated into synchronous firing of sets of neurons. At the motor end the code of the synfire chain has to be translated back into place and firing rate code. There is no physiological data to suggest how such translations are done.

Unfortunately, every experimental support for one of the three hypotheses could also be accounted for by the other hypotheses. It seems that at the present stage of knowledge and technique we must rely more on theoretical than on experimental considerations. In this respect the synfire hypothesis looks very attractive. It allows for the existence of a multitude of different processes in the same area, while the repertoire of modes that mass of cells can generate is relatively limited. It allows for interactions among processes which are difficult to explain in the dedicated line hypothesis. These interactions eliminate the need for a switchboard and a switchboard operator that connects the sensory analyzer with the motor executer as required by the dedicated line hypothesis. Above all the synfire hypothesis explains the need for the huge number of neurons and their extensive interconnections as found in the brain. It also suggests a clearcut mechanism by which synaptic strengthening may lay down a memory trace in the jungle of interconnections.

The main shortcoming of the synfire chain hypothesis relative to the dedicated line and mass action hypothesis is the inadequacy of the present research techniques for studying it. On one hand, there is no reason why synfire activity should be tightly locked to timing of external events, therefore, studies of PSTH of single units in response to external stimuli may be of little value for the study of the synfire chain. On the other hand, one would have to record from many thousands of units simultaneously before there is a good chance to observe such a synfire chain directly. The technology of recording has not yet reached the stage, although some microelectronic technology has been utilized for multi-electrode manufacturing (Pickard and Welberry 1976). Recently a way by which such multi-unit recording could be resolved into groups of synchronously activated neurons has been suggested by Gerstein et al. (1978).

Such techniques have still a long way to go before they could give direct evidence for the synfire hypothesis. Even if it were possible in the future to show directly that such chains evolve during learning and are activated during recall it would seem impossible to study the entire chain of any given process. Thus, we need not only new experimental techniques to show that synfire chains exist, but also a different approach for studying these processes. One such approach is the statistical analysis of the ECoG as suggested in this chapter.

10 Conclusion

It has been suggested that every physiologist would do justice to his readers if at the outset of his work he stated the prejudices he had while starting the work. This is perhaps too much to ask, but at least here in retrospect it would be fair to examine my own prenotions.

In the first place I believed that the spike trains carry the information processed by the brain. This is why the experiments described here were concentrated on microelectrode recordings. In addition I thought, like many others, that the important characteristic of information coding is the spatio-temporal organization of spikes in the population of neurons. This is the reason for devoting a considerable effort into developing a working multi-unit analyis hardware and improving the methods for statistical analysis. I also assumed that the nervous system is essentially a statistical machine. Neat organization and order are to be found when the average properties of nerve cell population are studied, while the detailed properties of individual neurons vary extensively around these average properties. My last prenotion was that the extensive network of connections among neurons has a function in the processing of information by the brain.

As is evident from the presentation in this book, the experimental results are in line with all these assumptions. Our understanding of these concepts was improved by the work presented here by quantifying the parameters of synaptic strength and cortical connectivity to the extent that the feasibility of various simple neural networks could be evaluated.

The main new outcome of the experiments described here is the idea of the synfire chain. The idea of organization of activity in synfire chains emerged because the observed, weak, synaptic connections would not explain the complex spatio-temporal sequences which were found occasionally in the three cells correlation.

Once the idea emerged it seemed to acquire life in its own right, because when assuming that at the higher brain levels the processing and transmission of information are indeed carried out by synfire chains we find numerous attractive properties that bring together the related aspects of anatomy, physiology, and psychophysics.

These properties are summarized in the concluding paragraphs:

a) *Limitless Variety.* The number of synfire chains is enormously large, since the number of ways by which cortical cells may be combined is almost limitless. Even if the processes are redundant and repeat themselves many times in different cortical regions there is still enough neuronal material to carry all the variety of mental activities and memories of the human mind.

b) *Resistance to Damage.* The synfire chain is very resistant to occasional fallout of its neurons. Adults lose about 100,000 neurons every day; but any appreciable loss of capability is noticable only in the long run.

c) *Memory Trace by Synaptic Strengthening.* The proper anatomical connections as required for a synfire chain exist only if the number of neurons per link is small, and the transition from a link size that can be supported by the intracortical connectivity to the size that cannot is very sharp (Fig. 24). That means that only if the synapses are strong enough to assure the synchronous transmission of activity between the links could the synfire chain function, and that there is again a very sharp transition between the synaptic strength that is sufficient to support a synfire arrangement and synaptic strength that is not. This property illustrates how enhanced synaptic efficiency may turn a nonfunctioning chain into a functioning one. The switchover is abrupt, supporting observations on animal and human learning in which there is a fast switchover from poor to good performance.

d) *Extensive Interconnectivity.* The synfire chains could be formed only in a matrix of very rich connectivity among the neurons. We are forced to postulate a huge connectivity even if we assume that only five cells are required to assure synchronous firing in the next link. When the synfire links are small enough, the cortex is full of potential synfire chains, that can become established when the appropriate combinations of synapses is strengthened. Development of such chains through experience proved to be much easier in the most extensively connected cortex — presumedly the human cortex.

e) *Neuron Morphology.* The unique nerve cell morphology of vertebrates in which all synaptic effects have first to converge into one region, the cell body, in order to trigger a spike is a prerequisite for the formation of synfire chains. The invertebrate neuropil in which the axon gives off several dendritic offshoots, each of which may have its own spike trigger zone, does not allow for enough combinations of inputs to support the development of synfire chains by experience.

f) *Switching.* The dependence of the synfire chain on the synaptic efficiency of its members makes it easy to turn such processes on and off by small changes in the excitability of neurons. Indeed in many recent studies of single-unit activity in behaving monkeys only small changes were found when attending to nonattending conditions were compared (e.g., Hocherman et al. 1976, Beaton and Miller 1975).

g) *Association.* If memory engrams are laid down in the form of synfire chains then the memory is also an associative memory. Synfire chains could support association due to the ability of partially activated links to regenerate full activity in the next stage. To illustrate this point let us assume that a certain concept is represented in the brain by activity along a certain synfire chain in which at each stage six neurons are firing synchronously. This synfire chain is mixed together with many other synfire chains whose activity represents other concepts. Concepts which are similar will be represented by synfire chains with partial overlaps at one or more links. As we enter this network of interlacing synfire chains with activity along one chain we reach a cross-over with another chain, in which we might face a situation where four of the six units of one chain belong also to a link of the other chain. If the total excitability of the region is increased so that now synchronous activity in four neurons will be enough to excite the neurons synchronously in the next link of the other chain, we shall find that one concept elicited another. Such associative connection is more likely to occur the more overlap there is between synfire chains representing the two concepts.

h) *Fine Discrimination.* Our ability to make fine sensory discrimination seems to require just the opposite process. Our ability to discriminate between two points of touch on our skin is much more refined than the receptive fields of the sensory fibers would suggest. Similarly, when we look at the verneir of a micrometer we are able to appreciate misalignment of 15 s of visual arc or less while the receptive fields of the nerve fibers in the optic nerve are several minutes of arc wide. Our ability to perceive a slight shift in a pitch of tone is about an order of magnitude better than the breadth of tuning of the fibers in the acoustic nerve. In the past it was suggested that successive stages of lateral inhibition (such as in Fig. 23B) could account for further refinement of the receptive fields. However, electrophysiological recordings from sensory cortices did not support the existence of such sharpening mechanisms. In fact, the receptive fields (for line) in the visual cortex are larger than the (circular) receptive fields in corresponding regions of the retina. Similarly, only 20% of the units in the auditory cortex have narrow tuning, and then they are not much narrower than the tuning of auditory nerve fibers (Abeles and Goldstein 1970).

An alternative hypothesis to the sharpening in space, which was not observed experimentally, is that sharpening occures in the time domain, that is by increased synchrony. In Fig. 31, we represent how synfire chains may separate overlapping stimuli without the need for refinement of receptive fields. Suppose stimulus B is activating synchronously the group of round cells (12, 13, 14) on the left. They in turn will activate the next group (cells 23, 24, 25) in synchrony and so on.

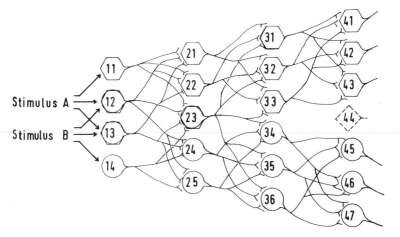

Fig. 31. Discrimination between overlapping activity by synfire chains

At the end of the network cells 45, 46 and 47 are activated synchronously representing the presence of stimulus B. When stimulus A is presented the "hexagonal" neurons (11, 12, 13) fire synchronously. Stimulus B is similar to stimulus A and therefore at that stage the units responding to the two patterns greatly overlap. At the next stage stimulus A is represented by the synchronous firing of cells 21, 22, and 23 and so on. At the end of the network stimulus A is represented by the synchronous firing of cells 41, 42, and 43.

This process of separation is not due to any sharp demarcation in threshold in the sense that exactly three synapses are enough to excite a neuron but two are not. Rather we assume that timing of firing at the next link when three synapses are activated, is more synchronous than the timing when two are activated. Cells 21 and 22 in Fig. 31 will fire also when stimulus B is presented, however their synchronization with cell 23 is not good enough to secure the activation of cells 31, 32 and 33 synchronously.

The succession of excitations down such a synfire chain may be compared to fractional distillation. There, at each higher stage the composition of the distillate becomes more pure. Here at successive stages down the line the separation between the stimuli improves because synchronous activity propagates securely while the subliminal firinge of partially excited neurons fails to propagate.

As stimuli A and B become more and more similar we shall need more and more stages to reach complete separation between the two stimuli. This might explain the lengthening of reaction time in psychophysical experiments where fine discrimination is required.

i) *Versatility.* How could the same network support on one occasion an expansion of activity into similar patterns while on other occasions it discriminates between very similar patterns? This would depend on the overall excitability of the neurons in the network. When the excitability is high we can have an associate expansion while if it is low we shall have refined discrimination.

j) *Interference.* When two synfire chains become active together and they share neurons in the same network they may destructively interfere with each other. Therefore, the synfire processing may be limited to one process at a time. This limitation is also true for many mental processes.

All these properties make the synfire chain a good candidate for the carrier of high-level processing in the brain. They are presented here in the hope that they shall stimulate further analysis on both theoretical and experimental levels.

Acknowledgements. It would not have been possible to carry out the various research projects reported here without the close collaboration of my students Y. Assaff, A. Arieli, R. Frostig, Y. Gottlieb, Y. Hodis and E. Vaadia; without the devoted technical help of V. Horn; and without the generous grants of: Hoffmann La Roche Co., The Rogoff Fund, The Hebrew University and Hadassah Fund, The Israel Center for Psychobiology, The Israel Commission for Basic Research, The Szold Foundation, The United States-Israel Binational Science Foundation, and The Israeli Ministry of Health Fund, to all of which I am very grateful.

My thanks are extended to C. Allweis, V. Braitenberg, M.H. Goldstein Jr., J. Magnes, G. Palm, and J. Rauschecker for reading the manuscript and making many useful suggestions, to V. Horn for her artwork and photography, to M. Sorotzkin and A. Shadmi for typing and retyping and retyping... the manuscript.

References

Abeles M (1981) The role of the cortical neuron: Integrator or coincidence detector. Isr J Med Sci (in press)

Abeles M (1982) Quantification of one, two and three cell correlations. (in preparation)

Abeles M, Goldstein MH Jr (1970) Functional architecture in cat primary auditory cortex: columnar organization and organization according to depth. J.Neurophysiol 33: 172-187

Abeles M, Goldstein MH Jr (1977) Multiple spike train analysis. Proc IEEE 65: 762-773

Abeles M, Lass Y (1975) Transmission of information by the axon. II: The channel capacity. Biol Cybernetics 19: 121-125

Beaton R, Miller JM (1975) Single cell activity in the auditory cortex of the unanesthetized, behaving monkey: Correlation with stimulus controlled behavior. Brain Res 100: 543-562

Beurle RL (1956) Properties of a mass of cells capable of regenerating pulses. Philos Trans R Soc London 240B: 55-94

Braitenberg V (1978a) Cortical architectonics: general and areal. In: Brazier MAB, Petche H (eds) Architectonics of the cerebral cortex. Raven Press, New York, pp 443-465

Braitenberg V (1978b) Cell assemblies in the cerebral cortex. In: Heim R, Palm G (eds) Theoretical approaches to complex systems, Lecture notes in biomathematics, Vol. 21. Springer, Berlin, Heidelberg, New York, pp 171-188

Braitenberg V (1981) Anatomical basis for divergence, convergence, and integration in the cerebral cortex. In: Grastyän E, Molnan P (eds) Sensory Function. Adv Physiol Sc. Vol. 16, pp 411-419

Burns DB, Webb AC (1979) The correlation between discharge times of neighboring neurons in isolated cerebral cortex. Proc R Soc London Ser B 203: 347-360

Cox DR (1970) Renewal theory. Methuen, London (1962) reprinted Science-paperbacks

Cragg BG (1975) The development of synapses in kitten visual cortex during visual deprivation. Exp Neurol 46: 445-451

Creutzfeldt OD (1974) The neuronal generation of the EEG. In: Handbook of electroencephalography and clinical neurophysiology, Vol. 2-C, Elsevier, Amsterdam, pp 5-55

Creutzfeldt OD (1978) The neocortical link: thoughts on the generality of structure and function of the neocortex. In: Brazier MAB, Petche H (eds) Architectonix of the cerebral cortex. Raven Press, New York, pp 357-383

Dickson JW, Gerstein GL (1974) Interactions between neurons in auditory cortex of the cat. J Neurophysiol 37: 1239-1261

Donchin E, Tueting P, Ritter W, Kutas M, Hefley E (1975) On the independence of the CNV and the P300 components of the human averaged evoked potential. Electroenephalogy, Clin Neurophysiol 38: 449-461

Eccles JC (1957) The Physiology of nerve cells. Johns Hopkins Press, Baltimore

Elul R (1972) The genesis of the EEG. Int Rev Neurobiol 15: 227-272

Erickson RP, Schiffman SS (1975) The chemical senses: a systematic approach. In: Gazzaniga MS, Blakemore C (eds) Handbook of psychobiology. Academic Press, New York, London, pp 393-426

Evans EF (1978) Place and time coding of frequency in the peripheral auditory system: some physiological pros and cons. Audiology 17: 369-420

Evans EF, Ross HF, Whitefield IC (1965) The spatial distribution of unit characteristic frequency in the primary auditory cortex of the cat. J Physiol (London) 179: 238-247

Fisken RA, Garey LJ, Powell TPS (1975) The intrinsic, association and commissural connections of area 17 of the visual cortex. Philos Trans R Soc London Ser B 272: 487-536

Freeman WJ (1975) Mass action in the nervous system. Academic Press, New York, London

Friedman DH (1968) Detection of signals by template matching. Johns Hopkins Press, Baltimore

Frostig R, Gottlieb Y, Vaadia E, Abeles M (1982) Local cortical networks: The effect of stimuli on activity and functional connectivity in the primary auditory cortex of cat. In preparation.

Gerstein GL, Perkel DH, Subramain KN (1978) Identification of functionally related neural assemblies. Brain Res 140: 43-62

Goldstein MH Jr (1968) Single unit studies of cortical coding of simple acoustic stimuli In: FD Carlson (ed) Physiological and biochemical aspects of nervous integration, Prentice-Hall, Englewood Cliffs, pp 131-151

Goldstein MH Jr, Abeles M (1975) Note on tonotopic organization of primary auditory cortex in the cat. Brain Res 100: 188-191

Goldstein MH Jr, Hall JL II, Butterfield BO (1968) Single unit activity in the primary auditory cortex of unanesthetized cats. J Acoust Soc Am 43: 444-455

Hartline HK, Wagner HG, Ratliff F (1956) Inhibition in the eye of limulus. J Gen Physiol 39: 651-673

Hebb DO (1944) The organization of behaviour: a neurophysiological theory. Wiley and Sous, New York

Hess R, Negishi K, Creutzfeldt O (1975) The horizontal spread of intracortical inhibition in the visual cortex. Exp Brain Res 22: 415-419

Hochermann S, Benson DA, Goldstein MH Jr, Heffner HE, Hienz RD (1976) Evoked unit activity in auditory cortex of monkeys performing a selective attention task. Brain Res 117: 51-68

Holden AV (1976) Models of the stochastic activity of neurons. Lecture notes in bio-mathematics, Vol. 12, Springer, Berlin, Heidelberg, New York

Hubel DH, Wiesel TN (1962) Receptive fields, binocular interaction and functional architecture in the cat's visual cortex. J Physiol 160: 106-154

Hubel DH, Wiesel TN (1979) Brain mechanisms of vision. Sci Am 241: 150-163

Imig TJ, Adrian HO (1977) Binaural columns in the primary field (A1) of cat auditory cortex. Brain Res 138: 241-257

John ER (1972) Switchboard versus statistical theories of learning and memory. Science 177: 850-864

John ER, Killiam KF (1960) Electrophysiological correlates of differential approach avoidance conditioning in the cat. J Nerv Ment Dis 131: 183-201

Kiang NY (1965) Stimulus coding in the auditory nerve and cochlear nucleus. Acta Oto-Laryngd 59: 186-200

Lorente de No R (1949) Cerebral cortex: architecture, intracortical connections, motor projection. In: Fulton JF (ed) Physiology of the nervous system, 3rd edn, Oxford Univ Press, New York, pp 288-312

Mather LH Jr, Mercer KL, Marshall DE (1978) Synaptic development in the rabbit superior colliculus and visual cortex. Exp Brain Res 33: 353-369

Merzenich MM, Knight PL, Roth GL (1975) Representation of cochlea within primary auditory cortex in the cat. J Neurophysiol 38: 231-249

Middlebrooks JC, Dykes RW, Merzenich MM (1980) Binaural response-specific bands in the primary auditory cortex (A1) of the cat: topographical organization orthogonal to isofrequency contours. Brain Res 181: 31-48

Miller GA (1963) The magical number seven, plus or minus two: some limits on our capacity for processing information. Psychol Rev 156: 81-97

Mitra NL (1955) Quantitative analysis of cells types in mammalian neocortex. J Anat 89: 467-483

Mitzdorf U, Singer W (1978) Prominent excitatory pathways in the cat visual cortex (A17 and A18): A current source density analysis of electrically evoked potentials. Exp Brain Res 33: 371-394

Mountcastle VB (1979) An organizing principle for cerebral function: the unit model and the distributed system. In: Edelman GM, Mountcastle VB (eds) The mindful brain. Cortical organization and the group selective theory of higher brain function. pp 7-50

Mountcastle VB, Lynch JC, Georgopoulos A, Sakata H, Acuna C (1975) Posterior parietal association cortex of the monkey: command functions for operations within extrapersonal space. J Neurophysiol 38: 871-908

Pandia DN, Hallet M, Mukherjee SK (1969) Intra and inter hemispheric connections of the neocortical auditory system in the rhesus monkey. Brain Res 14: 49-65

Perkel DH, Gerstein GL, Moore GP (1967a) Neuronal spike trains and stochastic point processes. I. The single spike train. Biophys J 7: 391-418

Perkel DH, Gerstein GL, Moore GP (1967b) Neuronal spike trains and stochastic point processes. II. Simultaneous spike trains. Biophys J 7: 419-440

Perkel DH, Gerstein GL, Smith MS, Tatton WG (1975) Nerve impulse patterns: A quantitative display technique for three neurons. Brain Res 100: 271-296

Pickard RS, Welberry TR (1976) Printed circuit microelectrodes and their application to honeybee brain. J Exp Biol 64: 39-44

Plonsey R (1977) Action potential sources and their volume conductor fields. Proc IEEE 65: 601-610

Rall W (1962) Electrophysiology of a dendritic neuron model. Biophys J 2: 145-167

Rall W (1967) Distinguishing theoretical synaptic potentials computed for different soma-dendritic distributions of synaptic input. J Neurophysiol 30: 1138-1168

Ribaupierre F de, Goldstein MH Jr, Yeni-Komshian G (1972) Intracellular study of the cat's primary auditory cortex. Brain Res 48: 185-204

Rolls ET (1978) Neurophysiology of feeding. Trens Neurosci 1: 1-3

Sampath G, Srinivasan SK (1977) Stochastic models for spike trains of single neurons. Lecture notes in biomathematics. Vol. 16, Springer, Berlin, Heidelberg, New York

Sherrington CS (1906) Integrative action of the nervous system. Yale Univ Press, New Haven

Sholl DA (1956) The organization of the cerebral cortex. Wiley and Sons, New York, p 49

Sousa-Pinto A (1973) Cortical projections of the medial geniculate body in the cat. Adv Anat Embryol Cell Biol 48: 1-42

Sutherland NS, Mackintosh NJ (1971) Mechanisms of animal discrimination learning. Academic Press, New York, London

Towe AL (1975) Notes on the hypothesis of columnar organization in somatosensory cerebral cortex. Brain Behav Evol 11: 16-47

Toyama K (1978) Interneuronal connectivity in cat visual cortex: studies by cross-correlation analysis of the response of two simultaneously recorded neurons. In: Integrative control function of the brain Ito M. (ed.) Vol. 1: 65-72 (ed.) Vol. 1: 65-72 Kodamsha Sci, Tokyo

Vaadia E, Gottlieb Y, Abeles M (1982) Single unit activity related to sensory-motor association in the auditory cortex of monkey. In preparation.

Walter WG (1964) Slow potential waves in the human brain associated with expectancy attention and decision. Arch Psychiatr Nervenkr 206: 309

Werner G, Mountcastle VB (1965) Neural activity in mechanoreceptive cutaneous afferents: stimulus, response relations, Weber funtions and information transmission. J Neurophysiol 28: 359-397

Young ED, Sachs MB (1979) Representation of steady-state vowels in the temporal aspects of the discharge patterns of populations of auditory-nerve fibers. J Acoust Soc Am 66: 1381-1403

Subject Index

A/σ amplitude 30
after potential 15
amplitude - mean squared 78, 80, 83, 84
association 93
asynchronous integration 25
auto-renewal density 12, 14, 15, 16, 18, 20, 60
average potential 78
axonal domain 36, 38

burst 18

cell assembly 65
code 72, 88
code - firing rate 89
coincidence 25, 68
columnar organization 33, 41
command neuron 85, 86, 87
common input 28, 29, 30, 33, 35, 37, 38, 47, 60, 62
concentric electrode 82
conductivity 22
connectivity 91, 92
connectivity - anatomical 36, 37, 49, 70
connectivity - measured 35, 37
contigent negative variation 88
cross-renewal density 12, 26, 28, 30, 32, 33, 46, 58, 60, 63, 68
current sink 5
current source 5

damage 73, 92
dedicated line 73, 75, 85, 86, 87, 89
dedicated line - definition 72
dendritic domain 36, 38
discrimination 93
discrimination reversal 52

electrocorticogram 6, 77, 78, 79, 80, 81, 82, 84, 88, 90
epileptic seizure 42, 46
excitability 11, 15, 20, 22

feature detector 86, 87
firing-asynchronous 68
firing pattern 13, 17
firing-periodic 16, 17, 18
firing rate 9, 11, 21

Gaussian probability 21, 22

information 10, 13
information code 11, 57, 85, 86, 91
information processing 91
information - transmission 71, 72, 74
inhibition 23, 30, 31. 32. 34. 37. 42, 49, 67
inhibition lateral 72, 93
integrator - neuron 68
interneuron 49, 63

learning 70, 90

macroelectrode 6, 78
map 33, 41, 72, 89
mass action 85, 86, 88, 89
medial geniculate body 47, 50
memory 93
memory trace 92
micripipete 8
microelectrode 6, 8, 91
mode of activity 16, 86
modulator 22
multi-unit activity 7

network 23, 30, 34, 35, 57, 65, 69, 70, 91

oscillation 14

pacemaker potential 15
parallel processing 73
Poisson process 14, 16, 23, 26, 67
population 78
positive 300 88
potential floctuations 21, 23, 24
Probability of firing 22

Studies of Brain Function

Coordinating Editor:
V. Braitenberg
Editors: **H. B. Barlow,**
H. Bullock, F. Florey,
O.-J. Grüsser, H. van der Loos

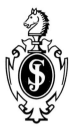

Springer-Verlag
Berlin
Heidelberg
New York

Volume 4
H. Braak

Architectonics of the Human Telencephalic Cortex

1980. 43 figures, 1 table. X, 147 pages
ISBN 3-540-10312-0

Contents: Introduction. – Types of Nerve Cells Forming the Telencephalic Cortex. – The Three Standard Techniques Used in Architectonics. – The Main Subdivisions of the Telencephalic Cortex. – The Allocortex. – The Proisocortex. – The Mature Isocortex. – Brain Maps. – Notes on Techniques. – References. – Subject Index.

Intended as an introduction to the architectonics of the human telencephalic cortex, this volume of **Studies of Brain Function** describes the prime nerve cell types of the cerebral cortex. A survey of technical methods available for use in architectonic studies is presented.
The main cerebral areas of both isocortex and the allocortex through the analysis of stained preparations of nerve cells, myelin sheaths, and pigment granules are examined in detail. Maps showing areas of the brain discussed are included. **Architectonics of the Human Telencephalic Cortex** is intended for advanced students and researchers in neurobiology.

Volume 5
H. Collewijn

The Oculomotor System of the Rabbit and Its Plasticity

1981. 128 figures. IX, 240 pages
ISBN 3-540-10678-2

The author of this monograph comprehensively describes his studies in the oculomotor system of the rabbit. This is in many respects a simplified model of the more complex system of visually more highly developed mammals, and its study has aided the understanding of eye movements in primates, including man. Main features are the analysis of optokinetics and vestibuloocular reflexes and their interaction, spontaneous oculomotor behavior, the processing and pathways of visual direction-selective signals and their relation to visually elicited eye movements.
Furthermore, the adaptability of the system is described according to physiological and pathological changes in stimulus conditions such as altered visuovestibular relations requiring recalibration of reflexes, dark-rearing, vestibular lesions and albinism. The emphasis is on pricise measurement of eye and head movements in restrained and freely moving animals, for which purpose new techniques were developed.
To illuminate the historical significance of rabbit oculomotor research in our understanding of eye movements, an English translation is included of Ter Braak's classical study of optokinetic nystagmus, first published in 1936, and still a source on inspiration today.

Springer-Verlag
Berlin
Heidelberg
New York